Keep fit for life

Meeting the nutritional needs
of older persons

**World Health
Organization**

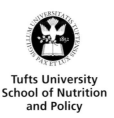

**Tufts University
School of Nutrition
and Policy**

WHO Library Cataloguing-in-Publication Data

Keep fit for life : meeting the nutritional needs of older persons.

    1.Aged 2.Aging – physiology 3.Nutrition 4.Nutritional requirements
    5.Nutritional status 6.Chronic disease – epidemiology 7.Social conditions
    8.Guidelines I.World Health Organization II.World Health Organization/
    Tufts University Consultation on Nutritional Guidelines for the Elderly
    (1998 : Boston, Mass.) III.Title: Meeting the nutritional needs of older persons

    ISBN 92 4 156210 2   (NLM classification: WT 115)

Designed by minimum graphics
Printed by Interprint Limited, Malta

Contents

Abbreviations & acronyms

ADH	Antidiuretic hormone
AVP	Arginine vasopressin
BMR	Basal metabolic rate
BIA	Bioelectrical impedance
BCM	Body cell mass
BMI	Body mass index
BUN	Blood urea nitrogen
CNCD	Chronic noncommunicable diseases
CHD	Coronary heart disease
DHA	Docosahexaenoic acid
DNA	Deoxyribonucleic acid
DTH	Delayed-type hypersensitivity (skin test)
EPA	Eicosaenoic acid
FAO	Food and Agriculture Organization of the United Nations
FWD	Free water deficit
IL-1	Interleukin-1
IL-2	Interleukin-2
IU	International units
NCD	Noncommunicable disease
NIDDM	Non-insulin-dependent diabetes mellitus
NK	Natural killer
NRS	Normal reference standards
1RM	One repetition maximum
PEM	Protein-energy malnutrition
Ppm	Parts per million
PUFA	Polyunsaturated fatty acids
RDA	Recommended daily allowance
RE	Retinol equivalents
RMR	Resting metabolic rate
RNA	Ribonucleic acid
WHO	World Health Organization
UNU	United Nations University
USDA	United States Department of Agriculture
VO2max	Maximal oxygen uptake

Foreword

The World Health Organization promotes health and well-being throughout the life course; this includes the attainment of the highest possible level of health and quality of life for the largest number of older persons, who are defined as people over 60 years of age.

In order to achieve the ultimate goal of healthy ageing and active ageing, WHO has developed a policy framework (Annex 1), which it introduced during the Second World Assembly on Ageing (Madrid, 8–12 April 2002). The framework focuses on such areas as:

- preventing and reducing the burden of disabilities, chronic disease and premature mortality;
- reducing the risk factors associated with noncommunicable diseases and functional decline as individuals age, while increasing factors that protect health;
- enacting policies and strategies that provide a continuum of care for people with chronic illness or disabilities;
- providing training and education to formal and informal carers;
- ensuring the protection, safety and dignity of ageing individuals;
- enabling people as they age to maintain their contribution to economic development, to activity in the formal and informal sectors, and to their communities and families.

Given the impact that good nutrition and keeping fit have on health and well-being in later life, WHO, in collaboration with the Tufts University USDA Human Nutrition Research Center on Aging, organized a consultation to review the scientific evidence linking diet and other factors—especially exercise—affecting nutritional status, disease prevention and health promotion for older persons (Boston, MA, 26–29 May 1998; see Annex 2 for list of participants). The consultation focused primarily on practical issues, including the establishment of explicit recommendations to improve the health and nutritional status of older persons in a wide variety of socioeconomic and cultural settings.

In this context, it is important to note that, despite the rapidly increasing proportion of older persons in the populations of developing countries, there is a scarcity of information concerning this group's specific nutritional needs.

Notwithstanding a deliberate effort to include relevant evidence in this volume wherever possible, the reality is that the majority of studies concerning older persons are still undertaken in industrialized countries. The degree of relevance of the information presented here remains to be verified by increased investigations in developing countries, which continue to be a high nutrition research priority.

During the production of a comprehensive report, representing the outcome both of the preparatory work and of the consultation itself, it was recognized that new information emerging in several key areas should also be included. The combined results presented here are intended as an authoritative source of information for nutritionists, general practitioners, gerontologists, medical faculties, nurses, care providers, schools of public health and social workers. The specific recommendations concerning nutrient intakes, food-based dietary guidelines, and exercise and physical activity should also interest a larger audience, including the general reader.

The main body discusses the epidemiological and social aspects of ageing, health and functional changes experienced with ageing, the impact of physical activity, assessment of the nutritional status of older persons, and nutritional guidelines for healthy ageing. Additional material covers food-based dietary guidelines for older adults (Annex 3)—with particular emphasis on healthy ageing and prevention of chronic noncommunicable diseases—and guidelines for promoting physical activity among older persons (Annex 4).

1. **Summary of recommendations**

1.1 **Nutrient intakes**

Nutrients for which reliable data are available directly from experiments conducted with older persons have been reviewed. Wherever possible, the recommendations that follow take into consideration not only the amount of a nutrient required to prevent a deficiency state but also a chronic disease. Additional studies are needed to determine the appropriate level of essential nutrients to maintain optimal immune response and to reduce the burden of disease.

- *Energy*

  1.4–1.8 multiples of the basal metabolic rate (BMR) to maintain body weight at different levels of physical activity.

- *Calcium*

  In addition to reducing fracture rates, 800–1200 mg/day (in the presence of adequate vitamin D nutrition) are beneficial for bone mineral density of the femur, neck and lumbar spine.

- *Copper*

  1.3–1.5 mg/day should be adequate for older persons.

- *Chromium*

  50 µg/day should achieve chromium balance in older persons.

- *Fat*

  30% in sedentary older persons and 35% for active older persons. Consumption of saturated fats should be minimized and not exceed 8% of energy.

- *Folate*

  400 µg/day have been shown to result in healthy homocysteine levels.

- *Iron*

  10 mg/day are adequate for older men and women assuming there are no excessive iron losses (e.g. from hookworm or schistosomiasis).

- *Magnesium*

  Dietary intakes of magnesium, which have been estimated in western countries to be between 225–280 mg/day, appear to be sufficient for individuals over the age of 65.

- *Protein*
  Generally speaking, protein intakes of 0.9–1.1 g/kg per day are beneficial for healthy older persons.

- *Riboflavin*
  Riboflavin requirements for older persons appear to be the same as for the young. The recommended daily allowance (RDA) is 1.3 mg for men and for 1.1 mg for women.

- *Selenium*
  50–70 µg/day should be more than adequate for older persons.

- *Vitamin A*
  600–700 µg retinol equivalents/day represent an adequate intake for older persons.

- *Vitamin B12*
  2.5 µg/day either from a vitamin B12 supplement or foods fortified with vitamin B12.

- *Vitamin C*
  Requirements for vitamin C are the same as for younger people; 60–100 mg/day appear to be adequate.

- *Vitamin D*
  10–15 µg/day are needed to ensure optimal bone health in older persons.

- *Vitamin E*
  100–400 IU/day have been shown to reduce recurrent cardiovascular disease.

- *Vitamin K*
  60–90 mg/day are an adequate intake for older persons.

- *Zinc*
  Required intake for dietary zinc in people over 65:

High Zn availability (50+%)	Men	4.2 mg/day
	Women	3.0 mg/day
Moderate Zn availability (30%)	Men	7.0 mg/day
	Women	4.9 mg/day
Low Zn availability (15%)	Men	14.0 mg/day
	Women	9.8 mg/day

1.2 **Food-based dietary guidelines**

It is clear that a wide variety of food cultures and cuisines can promote healthy ageing. The nutrient-based approach to recommended intakes is limited in that it does not consider the environmental, socioeconomic and lifestyle context of eating. Nor does it adequately address the chemical complexity of foods and the interaction and synergies, whether between foods or individual food components.

In 1996 FAO and WHO jointly organized a consultation on the development of food-based dietary guidelines as part of the two organizations' continuing efforts to increase the relevance and effectiveness of nutritional recommendations in everyday life. This method takes into account diet and health relationships in a culturally sensitive manner, thereby providing consumers with easier ways to make healthy food choices (see Annex 3 for a detailed discussion of food-based dietary guidelines for older adults).

The main recommendations, using the food-based dietary guideline approach, are as follows.

- Emphasize healthy traditional vegetable- and legume-based dishes.
- Limit traditional dishes/foods that are heavily preserved/pickled in salt and encourage the use of herbs and spices.
- Introduce healthy traditional foods or dishes from other cuisines (e.g. tofu in Europe and the tomato in Asia).
- Select nutrient-dense foods such as fish, lean meat, liver, eggs, soy products (e.g. tofu and tempeh) and low-fat dairy products, yeast-based products (e.g. spreads), fruits and vegetables, herbs and spices, whole-grain cereals, nuts and seeds.
- Consume fat from whole foods such as nuts, seeds, beans, olives and fatty fish. Where refined fats are necessary for cooking, select from a variety of liquid oils, including those high in ω-3 and ω-9 fats. Avoid fatty spreads.
- Enjoy food and eating in the company of others. Avoid the regular use of celebratory foods (e.g. ice cream, cakes and pastries in western culture, confectioneries and candies in Malay culture, and crackling pork in Chinese culture).
- Encourage the food industry and fast-food chains to produce ready-made meals that are low in animal fats.
- Eat several (5–6) small non-fatty meals. This pattern appears to be associated with greater food variety and lower body fat and blood glucose and lipid levels, especially if larger meals are eaten early in the day.
- Transfer as much as possible of one's food culture, health knowledge and related skills to one's children, grandchildren and the wider community.

- Be physically active on a regular basis and include exercises that strengthen muscles and improve balance.
- Avoid dehydration by regularly consuming, especially in warm climates, fluids and foods with a high water content.

1.3 Phytochemicals

In addition to the recognized essential nutrients, there are many other food components about which little is known; they nevertheless can have important—e.g. anti-inflammatory, anti-microbial, anti-oxidant, anti-mutagenic, anti-angiogenic or hormonal—biological effects, capable of lowering the risk of major health problems such as cancer and heart disease. It is thus important to obtain essential nutrients through a food-based approach rather than depending on vitamin and mineral supplements. High priority should be given to research into identifying the presence and role of these phytochemicals in the diets of older person. The potential health-promoting aspects of food components should also be carefully considered in formulating agricultural and trade policies and strategies.

1.4 Water intake

Many degenerative age-related diseases aggravate the tendency towards dehydration in older persons. In addition, dehydration is a common complication of acute illness in this population group. As a rule of thumb, adults require about 30 ml/kg of water per day. However, this intake level may be insufficient to meet the fluid needs of underweight adults. An alternative approach is to provide 100 ml/kg for the first 10 kg, 50 ml/kg for the next 10 kg and 15 ml/kg for the remaining weight. Unless there is renal failure or some other reason to restrict intake, even underweight adults should receive at least 1500 ml of fluid per day.

1.5 Exercise and physical activity

No group can benefit more than older persons from regularly performed exercise. Aerobic exercise has long been an important recommendation for preventing and treating many of the chronic and typically age-associated diseases, including non-insulin-dependent diabetes mellitus (NIDDM), hypertension, heart disease and osteoporosis. Moreover, research indicates that strength training is necessary both to stop or reverse sarcopenia—the age-associated loss of body protein—and to increase bone density. Increasing muscle strength and muscle mass in older persons is a realistic strategy for maintaining this group's functional status and independence. The following recommendations for aerobic and strength-training exercises are appropriate for individuals age 60 and older. Any exercise programme should, of course, always first be discussed with one's health care provider.

1.5.1 *Aerobic exercise*

Older persons should build up to at least 30 minutes of aerobic exercise—for example walking, swimming, aqua gym and stationary cycling—on most, if not all, days.

1.5.2 *Strength training*

Strength training 2 to 3 days a week, with a day of rest between workouts, is recommended to maintain bone and muscle strength.

2. Epidemiological and social aspects of ageing

2.1 Demography *(1)*

There are an estimated 605 million older persons, i.e. age 60 and over, in the world today, nearly 400 million of whom live in low-income countries. Greece and Italy have the highest proportion of older persons (both 24% in 2000). By 2025, the number of older persons worldwide is expected to reach more than 1.2 billion, with about 840 million of these in low-income countries. Within the next 25 years, Europe is projected to retain its title as the world's oldest region. Older persons currently represent around 20% of the total population and the proportion is expected to increase to 29% by 2025.

By 2025 Japan and Switzerland will have the highest proportion of older persons (35%), followed (in decreasing order) by Italy, Germany, Greece and Spain (all > 30%). By 2025, the proportion of the population aged 60 and over is expected to reach 25% in North America, 21% in eastern Asia, 14% in Latin America and the Caribbean, and 11% in south and central Asia. During the next 25 years, many low-income countries will displace high-income countries in terms of the number of people aged 60 and over. By 2025, five low-income countries will be among the ten countries with the largest population of older persons in the world: China (287 million), India (168 million), Indonesia (35 million), Brazil (33 million), and Pakistan (18 million).

The most dramatic changes are found in the oldest age group (80 years and over). In Europe alone, it is estimated that this population will grow from 21.4 million in 2000 to 35.7 million in 2025. The proportion of centenarians in high-income countries also continues to grow; presently, it exceeds one in every thousand people.

With the exception of those countries where female mortality is high during infancy and the reproductive years and overall life expectancy is short, many of the oldest group will be women. For example, in Europe there are 15.2 million women aged 80 and above compared to only 6.2 million men (virtually doubling—from 7.2 million women and 3.3 million men aged 80 and above *(2)*—since 1970). In 1900, the North American/European sex-based difference in life expectancy was typically 2 to 3 years. Currently, women in most high-income countries outlive men by 5 to 9 years. Women today have lower mortality than men do in every age group and for most causes of death. In 2000, average female life expectancy at birth exceeded 80 years in 30 countries, and it is approaching this threshold in many others. While the sex differential in life expectancy is usually smaller in low-income countries, between 2000 and 2025 both the proportion and number of older women aged 60 are expected to soar from 170 million to 373 million in Asia, and from 22 million to 46 million in Africa.

2.2 **Reasons for population ageing**

Mortality rates have declined in virtually all countries due to progress in preventing infectious diseases and improving hygiene, sanitation and overall social development and living standards. As a result, average life expectancy at birth in low-income countries rose from around 45 years in the early 1950s to 64 years in 1990. The average life expectancy throughout the world is projected to reach 73 years in 2020. While life expectancy, even in the richest countries, was no higher than 50 years at the beginning of the 20th century, today it is more than 75 years. Countries such as China, Honduras, Indonesia and Viet Nam have added 25 years to life expectancy at birth in just four decades. In contrast, it took 114 years—from 1865 to 1980—for the population of older persons in France to double from 7% to 14% of the total.

This decline in mortality was accompanied more recently by an equally sharp fall in birth rates, the only exception being most of sub-Saharan Africa. For instance, total fertility rates in China declined from 5.5 in 1970 to 1.8 currently; respective figures are 5.1 and 2.2 for Brazil, and 5.9 and 3.1 for India. Ultimately, the demographic transition leading to population ageing can be summarized as a shift from high mortality/high fertility to low mortality/low fertility.

As fertility declines and more people live longer, the relative weight of society's main dependent groups—children and older persons—is shifting towards older persons. While the total dependency ratio (defined as the number of young people aged 0–14 years plus persons aged 60 and older divided by the population of working persons aged 15–59) may in fact be declining, the old-age dependency ratio (defined as the number of persons aged 60 and over divided by the population of working age 15–59 years) will continue to exhibit steady increases. The claim that older persons use more public resources than young dependants is the subject of considerable debate. Nevertheless, the weight of the old component of the total dependency ratio has considerable economic significance.

For example, by 2025 there will be about 32 older people in East Asia for every 100 working-age persons (Table 1). In terms of economic dependency in this region of everyone older than 45 (defined as all people 45 years of age and over who are not wage-earners), by 2025 there will be 40 people economically dependent on 100 working people. Such a large dependency ratio requires policy responses to improve the health of older persons, thereby increasing their ability to contribute longer to the larger society.

Table 1. **Dependency ratios (%) for East Asia, 1975 and 2025**[a]

	1975	2025
Age dependency (60+)	15	32
Economically dependent population (45+)	18	40

[a] *Source: reference 1.*

2.3 Improvements in biological age

While the average age of populations is clearly increasing, evidence of improvements in biological age at a given chronological age, especially in high-income countries, should also be factored in (3, 4). The most recent findings for some high-income countries show that severe disability is declining in older people at a rate of 1.5% per year. In the United Kingdom of Great Britain and Northern Ireland, for example, the percentage of disabled older people fell between 1976 and 1994. If current trends continue, it is estimated that by 2050 the percentage will have decreased by half of 1994 levels (Figure 1).

As populations in both low- and high-income countries age, it becomes more apparent that investments in ageing and health, including nutrition, have potentially huge pay-offs. Ensuring that older persons continue to contribute productively to society as workers, volunteers and providers instead of being only recipients of care and services enhances their social and economic involvement and overall well-being. In addition, fewer resources will be required to sustain them during their final years. However, remaining self-reliant and productive depends on continuing good health. Individuals, therefore, have to take greater responsibility for their health and adopt health-enhancing lifestyles that include healthy eating and adequate exercise. In short, they need to embrace the notion of healthy ageing.

2.4 Health status of older persons

With the increase in life expectancy occurring in high-income countries since the beginning of this century, leading causes of death have shifted dramatically from infectious to noncommunicable diseases and from younger to older individuals. In industrialized countries, about 75% of deaths in people over the age of 65 are now from heart disease, cancer and cerebrovascular disease. In contrast, at the turn of the century, infectious disease was responsible for 50% of deaths, while heart disease, cancer and stroke combined contributed to only 35% of deaths. Public health measures have had major positive effects in increasing life expectancy from birth. In addition, a significant portion of the decline in mortality observed since 1960 has been the postponement of death from chronic diseases. Life expectancy at age 60, or even 85, is also rapidly improving.

Figure 1. **Percentage, by age, of men unable to perform four activities of daily living in 1976, 1987 and 1994ᵃ**

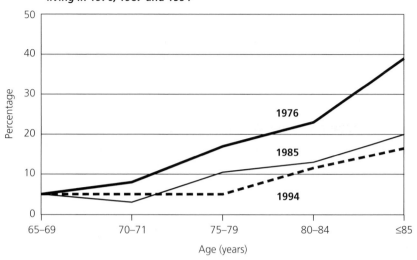

ᵃ *Reproduced from reference 4 with the permission of the publisher.*

Similarly, as populations age in low-income countries, the main causes of death previously associated with premature deaths at early ages lose their pre-eminence and are gradually replaced by causes of death more typically associated with high-income countries. For instance, in Latin America the estimated change between 1970 and 2015 in the proportional contribution of the three most common causes of death is as follows: infectious diseases, 33.4% to 9.3%; circulatory diseases, 8.9% to 10.8%; and neoplasms, 7.2% to 16.9% (5).

As in high-income countries, ischaemic heart disease and cerebrovascular diseases followed by neoplasms and respiratory diseases, now cause the vast majority of deaths occurring at older ages in low-income countries. Mortality figures can be deceptive, however, by creating the impression that the diseases of the past no longer prevail. Morbidity figures are more useful since, while they indicate that many diseases no longer kill as early in life, it is nevertheless clear that they are still prevalent. For the foreseeable future low-income countries will continue to face the dual challenge of coping with both high morbidity and disability rates due to infectious diseases and high rates for the superimposed emerging chronic diseases characteristic of ageing societies.

2.5 **Functioning and disability**

As people age, there tends to be a concomitant increase in the presence and number of chronic conditions together with a greater dependence on caretakers. Generally speaking, people are regarded as dependent if they need help to perform basic daily tasks, and their level of functioning is often assessed accordingly. Large-scale, cross-national comparisons of dependency ratio prevalence present conceptual and methodological difficulties since they need to be evaluated against different social, cultural, physical and environmental factors. Even if there is an appreciable margin for methodological error, comparisons in Asia (*6*) and Europe (*7*) reveal wide differences between communities in the performance of these basic daily tasks. WHO has released a new version of the International Classification of Functioning, Disability and Health (ICF) (*8*). The aim is to provide a unified and standard language and framework for the description of human functioning and disability in relevant health and health-related domains.

Obvious questions that arise include who assists dependent older persons and who bears the cost. Assistance may be in the form of informal help from family, neighbours and friends, or formal long-term care involving a series of medical and social services. Data show that in the vast majority of cases, as ageing proceeds women are more likely to be both caregivers and care recipients. The challenge is to develop prevention programmes that address the important sex-based differences that occur in the health status of older persons.

2.5.1 *Coronary heart disease and stroke*
Coronary heart disease and stroke have become the major causes of death and disability among both ageing women and men. They account for close to 60% of all adult female deaths in a typical high-income country and are also the major cause of death among women aged 50 and above in low-income countries. However, women are typically ten years older than men when they experience symptoms of heart disease, and they may be up to 20 years older before they experience their first heart attack. Heart disease and stroke are nevertheless still commonly considered men's health problems.

2.5.2 *Cancer*
The five most deadly cancers worldwide are also the most common in terms of their incidence. Together they account for about 50% of all cancer cases and deaths. Among men, the leading eight killer sites are lung, stomach, liver, colon-rectum, oesophagus, mouth/pharynx, prostate and lymph nodes. In women, the leading killer sites are breast, stomach, colon-rectum, cervix, lung, ovary, oesophagus and liver. Analysis of the risk factors involved in the development of major cancers shows that a few such factors dominate—tobacco, diet, alcohol, infections and hormones; fortunately, *all* lend themselves to preventive action.

2.5.3 *Osteoporosis and bone fractures*
Osteoporosis and associated bone fractures are one of the major causes of disability and death that result in enormous medical expense the world over. It is estimated that the number of hip fractures worldwide will rise from 1.7 million in 1990 to

around 6.3 million by 2050. Women are more prone because their bone loss accelerates after menopause. Factors such as diet, physical activity and smoking are closely associated with osteoporosis. Lifestyle modifications, particularly increased calcium intake and physical activity, could over time have an important preventive impact on fracture rates.

2.6 Nutrition problems in low-income countries

The nutritional status of older persons in low-income countries is inadequately documented. Logistical difficulties and the absence of simple, easy-to-handle assessment instruments compound data-collection problems in this environment. As a result, nutritional data for older adults are inadequate. The scanty, mainly hospital-based, data that are available are hardly comprehensive, and they fail to incorporate essential indicators of nutritional status.

Food-intake assessments are rarely conducted among older persons in low-income countries, yet such assessments play a crucial role in detecting relationships between dietary exposure and disease causation. Nutritional problems are at the root of the major communicable and chronic noncommunicable diseases, which are impediments to achieving both national and international health goals and economic and social progress.

2.7 Malnutrition and food security

Malnutrition in low-income countries is closely related to household food security—the ability to produce or buy adequate, safe and good-quality food to meet the dietary requirements of all members at all times. Many households in low-income countries, and some pockets in high-income countries, experience transitory and chronic food insecurity. Causes of food insecurity are numerous including erratic weather, rapid population growth, high food prices, and changing agricultural practices and eating habits. Other factors include poor food distribution and marketing systems, low purchasing power, inadequate research and extension support for indigenous food crops, lack of appropriate technologies to enhance food production and processing, and inadequate mechanisms for dealing with emergency food situations. At the household level, the effects of protracted drought and the harsh socioeconomic impact characterizing some low-income countries continue to adversely affect household food availability and accessibility, thus ensuring that certain sections of the population remain malnourished due to low food intakes.

Undernutrition is a global problem that is usually caused by a lack of food or a limited range of foods that provide inadequate amounts of specific nutrients or other food components, e.g. protein, dietary fibre and micronutrients. Excessive intake of food or specific forms of food may also be harmful. Malnutrition among older persons can occur in economically disadvantaged groups even within privileged societies, and in pockets of poverty or social isolation. Reasons for undernutrition include decreased food availability and affordability; lack of interest or awareness affecting intake; malabsorption or increased nutrient requirements; and traditional habits or beliefs whether of the elderly or their caretakers.

Older persons are vulnerable to protein-energy malnutrition (PEM), which is one of the main public health problems in most low-income tropical and subtropical countries with predominantly rural populations. Since PEM may not be as obvious in this population group due to changes in body composition related to age, some observers suggest that it may be more appropriate to talk about protein-energy dysnutrition in older persons (9). The underlying causes of malnutrition in low-income countries are not so much lack of food as limited knowledge and traditional views about what older persons should or should not eat. Migration of elders and/or of their younger counterparts may also play a role in worsening malnutrition among older persons due to the negative impact on traditional social support structures.

Older persons in these environments may also over-eat the wrong foods. The result is an increasingly common global paradox, the concurrent presence of chronic diseases such as obesity, diabetes, cancer and other chronic illnesses associated with combined forms of undernutrition. By 2020 all these problems may well be further compounded if old-age dependency ratios worsen, even in low-income countries which currently have generally favourable ratios. There may be increased competition for resources as the growing numbers of older persons join other groups that are vulnerable to nutritional deficiencies, for example under-five children, pregnant and lactating women, street children, displaced persons/refugees, and female heads of household.

2.8 Government response to ageing populations

High-income countries have been adjusting for some time to meeting the needs of their older citizens. In contrast, most governments of densely populated low-income countries are only just beginning to recognize the long-term socioeconomic implications of their ageing populations. They are starting to examine factors affecting the care and quality of life of older persons, including the impact of the weakening of traditional joint family systems, the absence of social protection schemes and the rural-to-urban migration of younger people. In response, governments are seeking to develop national policies and strategies for dealing with the emerging multiple age-related social, economic and health challenges across society. Indeed, ageing is starting to be viewed as an important development issue.

2.9 Prevention of chronic disease at every stage of life

Prospects for healthy ageing are affected by nutrition at every stage of life. A pregnant woman requires adequate nutrition because fetal malnutrition and low birth weight can lead to increased risk of chronic diseases such as hypertension, coronary heart disease, adult onset diabetes and autoimmune thyroid disease (10–13). Malnutrition during infancy can also contribute to these consequences. Fetal iodine deficiency and iron deficiency in early childhood can have lasting consequences for cognitive development. The risk of osteoporosis at an older age is strongly influenced by bone density at puberty based on adequacy of calcium and vitamin D intake in childhood and by the adequacy of these nutrients throughout life (14). Regardless of predisposing factors, dietary and other environmental factors influence morbidity and mortality at every age. Because of the cumulative effect of adverse factors throughout life, it is particularly important for older persons to adopt dietary and lifestyle practices that minimize further risk of ill-health and maximize their prospects for healthy ageing.

Prevention of chronic disease through proper nutrition plays a significant role in each phase of prevention.

- *Primary prevention* involves risk-factor modification to prevent the occurrence of disease, for example by increasing dietary fibre and reducing animal fat intakes to diminish the incidence of colorectal cancer.

- *Secondary prevention* involves screening for a disease before it becomes symptomatic, for example routine use of serum cholesterol testing to assess risk of coronary heart disease (CHD) combined with appropriate follow-up intervention, for example decreasing intake of animal fats or increasing intake of plant foods.

- *Tertiary prevention* involves treating and minimizing the complications of a disease once it has occurred, for example reducing the risk for a future coronary event by eating fish weekly and increasing intake of antioxidant sources, including larger quantities of a particular variety of fruits and vegetables and possibly antioxidant supplements.

While nutritional interventions have been shown to be effective in terms of primary and secondary prevention, changes in dietary patterns early in life are likely to be even more beneficial. As a first step, an individual's dietary patterns should be identified. Where diagnostic capabilities are available, appropriate and affordable, a health practitioner can also identify early features of chronic disease and offer nutritional advice and support, for example for older adults with abdominal obesity, glucose intolerance, hypertension or dyslipidaemias.

As awareness of preventive nutrition measures increases, premature deaths related to chronic diseases should decrease. The leading causes of death associated with diet include coronary heart disease, stroke, cancer, diabetes, influenza and other infectious diseases. Furthermore, alcohol consumption is strongly associated with suicide, accidental injury and chronic liver disease. Several other diseases derived substantially from lifestyle factors contribute significantly to morbidity and mortality and are indirectly linked to nutrition. For example, obesity aggravates chronic obstructive pulmonary diseases such as chronic bronchitis, and emphysema induced by smoking and air pollutants. Moreover, these patients are often malnourished, further promoting decline of pulmonary function and increasing mortality.

The rising prevalence of chronic diseases in ageing populations is a substantial burden not only for health care systems but also for social and family structures due to dependency resulting from osteoporotic fractures, visual impairment, arthritic immobility and vascular or other dementias. Scientific advances are gradually uncovering nutritional components of many of these problems.

2.10 Nutritional components in chronic diseases

2.10.1 *Coronary heart disease*

Proper food intake, particularly reduced intake of total and saturated fat and increased intake of plant food, is a cornerstone in preventing and managing coronary risk factors, notably lipoprotein disorders, and protecting against arterial damage, whether by oxidation or other means. A number of food factors may afford cardio-protection through various pathways such as endothelial function, platelet aggregation, blood pressure, homocysteinaemia and cardiac membrane electrical stability. Candidate food factors include micronutrients such as folate and vitamins B6 and B12, which lower homocysteine levels; *n*-3 fatty acids, which decrease platelet aggregation and arrhythmogenesis; and vitamins C and E and phytochemicals, which are antioxidants for lipoprotein, deoxyribonucleic acid (DNA) and all cell membrane phospholipids.

2.10.2 *Cancer*

A high intake of total fat increases the risk of some types of cancer—perhaps cancer of the breast (if very low-fat populations are included in the analyses), almost certainly of the colon, and possibly of the prostate, rectum and ovaries. Other dietary factors, including intake of alcohol; charred, smoked, and salt- and nitrate-cured foods; and naturally occurring contaminants such as aflatoxins and N-nitroso compounds also pose a potential risk for cancer.

Food-intake patterns emphasizing unrefined foods high in dietary fibre are associated with low rates of certain cancers, especially of the breast and colon. Fruits and green and yellow vegetables, which are important sources of antioxidant vitamins, putative chemo-preventive phytochemicals such as phenols and indoles, and dietary fibre are also associated with reduced risk of several forms of cancer. For example, high intakes of β-carotene from food appear to reduce the incidence of cancer of the lung, breast, oral mucosa, bladder and oesophagus.In contrast, β-carotene supplements may actually increase cancer risk among smokers (*15*).

Vitamin C appears to have a protective effect against oesophageal, stomach, cervical, breast and lung cancers. Low intakes of vitamin E are correlated with increased risk of cancer in several organs, while there is evidence suggesting that calcium and selenium protect against cancer. Where primary prevention is concerned, several studies have demonstrated that diet can have a beneficial effect on pre-cancerous lesions, for example colonic adenoma (*16*).

2.10.3 **Stroke**

Animal fat, saturated fatty acids and total fat intakes have been positively related to the risk of cerebral infarct in some, though not all, studies, whereas they are inversely correlated with the incidence of cerebral haemorrhage. Recently, poor blood concentrations of folate and vitamin B6 and high concentrations of plasma homocysteine have been linked to an increased risk of extracranial carotid-artery stenosis in older adults, thus suggesting an important role for these two vitamins in stroke prevention. Many observers consider that plant-derived foods may protect against stroke, probably for several reasons including by lowering blood pressure. Vitamin E has been associated with a reduced risk of ischaemic stroke but an increased risk of haemorrhaegic stroke. Alcohol increases stroke risk in a linear fashion.

2.10.4 **Non-insulin-dependent diabetes mellitus**

Body fat and its abdominal distribution are consistently related to the prevalence of Type II diabetes whereas diet, weight loss and exercise, which can normalize blood sugars in most patients, appear to delay the onset of diabetic sequelae (*17*). Cohort studies demonstrate an interaction between total glycaemic load (unfavourable) and cereal-derived dietary fibre (favourable) in the prediction of NIDDM development (*18, 19*). People with diabetes are generally counselled to consume small quantities of food more frequently in place of large meals, to select low-glycaemic index foods, and to eat small amounts of animal fat while selecting high nutrient density foods (*20*). Essential micronutrients may be marginal as the pathogenesis of diabetes proceeds, e.g. *n*-3 fatty acids (*19, 21*), vitamin E (*22*), chromium (*23*) and magnesium (*18*) acting through insulin action or glucose handling.

2.10.5 **Osteoporosis**

There is substantial evidence that calcium and vitamin D protect against osteoporosis. High calcium intake during the early years contributes to greater peak bone mass. During the later years, calcium, together with vitamin D, prevents negative calcium balance and reduces the rate of bone loss. However, due to the limitations of observational research, there is a lack of concordance in epidemiological studies associating calcium and vitamin D intake and fracture risk. Nevertheless, clinical trials with daily supplements of these nutrients clearly demonstrate a significant reduction in the rate of age-related bone loss and secondary hyperparathyroidism and the incidence of fractures, especially of the hip. In addition to calcium, other minerals including boron, copper, magnesium, manganese and zinc appear to contribute to the maintenance of bone density with age. Sodium adversely affects calcium balance through the promotion of urinary calcium loss (24). There is increasing evidence that phytoestrogens from soy and some other plant sources may account for better bone health than might otherwise be expected for a given calcium intake (25), with effects mediated via the β-estrogen receptor (26). Other nutrients such as vitamin K, through osteocalcin, and essential fatty acids also contribute to bone health. Although they are not as well established, dietary risk factors for osteoporosis include excess consumption of caffeine, protein and alcohol (14). Thus, as in other chronic noncommunicable diseases, an overall food pattern is likely to be more important for bone health among older persons than any single food factor taken alone.

2.10.6 *Other chronic conditions*

A growing body of evidence suggests that preventive nutrition strategies may also play a significant role in other chronic conditions which, while not necessarily directly associated with risk of fatality, do affect independence, quality of life and health care expenditure. For example, studies have demonstrated that supplementation with antioxidant vitamins, vitamin B6, zinc and/or multivitamin/ mineral formulations can enhance *immune response* in older persons, and that this action appears to be associated with reduced risk and duration of infectious disease episodes. Obesity exacerbates conditions such as rheumatoid arthritis, and particularly osteoarthritis, which are highly prevalent among older persons. Recent evidence suggests a beneficial effect on both pathogenesis and clinical signs as a result of an increased intake of several micronutrients (27, 28).

Accumulating evidence also suggests an important relationship between the incidence of age-related cataract and nutritional status, particularly where the antioxidant vitamins C and E are concerned. In two prospective randomized clinical trials conducted in China, supplementation with a multivitamin preparation or a riboflavin/niacin formula was found to significantly reduce the prevalence of nuclear cataract in older subjects relative to placebo controls. Recently, epidemiological studies have indicated an inverse association between generous intakes of dietary carotenoids (especially lutein and zeaxanthin from foods such as corn and eggs) and vitamins C and E with the incidence of age-related *macular degeneration*, which is the leading cause of irreversible blindness among older adults (29, 30).

Several studies suggest that mild or subclinical vitamin deficiency in free-living populations play a role in the pathogenesis of declining *neurocognitive function* with age. Healthy older adults with low blood levels of some vitamins—particularly folate, vitamin B12, vitamin C and riboflavin—have been found to score poorly on tests of memory and non-verbal abstract thinking. Significant correlations have also been reported between poor indices of thiamine, riboflavin and iron nutriture and impaired cognitive performance and electroencephalographic indices of neuropsychological function. The inverse correlation between plasma homocysteine levels and carotid artery stenosis suggests that low B-vitamin status may be related to the risk of cerebrovascular disease with its associated changes in cognitive function. High-dose vitamin E supplementation appears to delay the progression of Alzheimer disease, although scientists have not yet identified why vitamin E, other antioxidants and other food factors may have an effect on the illness.

3. Health and functional changes with ageing

Ageing is associated with a decline in many body functions, an accompanying change in structure, loss of lean mass and a relative increase in fat mass over time (*31*). Research over the past several decades has progressively reduced the number of these changes considered to be intrinsically due to ageing while it has increased those that are attributed to age-related disuse, inactivity and degenerative diseases (*32*). Thus, for example, whereas cardiac dilatation is no longer ascribed to ageing *per se* but is rather considered a result of age-related hypertension, the decline in peak heart rate continues to be attributed to ageing. In reality, it is impossible to distinguish fully between the health effects of age-related illness and ageing itself. Unless otherwise noted, the data reviewed below are from studies performed among healthy older adults in high-income countries. Data on nutrient effects on chronic disease are described separately.

3.1 Physical changes

3.1.1 *Body weight*

Studies on normative populations in high-income countries demonstrate that body weight increases during adult life until 50–59 years, after which it declines (*33*). In agrarian societies, weight seems to be more stable until age 60 and then declines over the next two decades.

3.1.2 *Protein and muscle*

Some of the most dramatic changes seen with age are in body composition. Lean body mass declines over the adult age span and accelerates beyond age 80. While the average woman's lean body mass is always less than a man's, the decline is just as striking; it places older women closer to the threshold below which loss of lean tissue begins to have overt clinical consequences. Some studies show accelerated decline after menopause, suggesting a role for estrogen in the maintenance of lean tissue other than bone. The condition or state of sarcopenia (3.1.4) strongly influences muscle strength, gait and balance, while it contributes to the risk of falls and frailty in older persons.

This age-related change is even more dramatic if the decline is expressed in terms of muscle mass instead of total lean body mass. Twenty-four-hour creatinine excretion was assessed as a measure of muscle mass in a cross-sectional study of

959 healthy men aged 20 to 97 years from the Baltimore Longitudinal Study on Aging cohort. The decline by decade was found to be particularly dramatic after age 60. Direct regional assessments of skeletal muscle cross-sectional area can be made using image analysis of computed tomography scans of the area of interest. At the level of the mid-thigh, for example, muscle accounts for 90% of the cross-sectional area in active young men but only 30% of the area in frail older women.

3.1.3 *Decline in body cell mass*

Fat-free mass consists of body cell mass (BCM), extracellular fluid and the extracellular solids such as collagen and bone mineral. BCM can be further compartmentalized into the fat-free portion of cells within muscle, viscera and the immune system. Although the available direct evidence is limited, most researchers in body composition agree that BCM is the functionally important compartment for determining energy expenditure, protein needs and the metabolic response to physiologic stress (the acute phase response). Further functional consequences are implicit in the BCM subcompartments—muscle BCM directly predicts strength and thus functional status (34), visceral and muscle BCM is the major determinant of energy needs (35), and immune function depends on an adequately constituted immunocompetent cell system. A key observation made by Krieger (36), and later more comprehensively—and tragically—by the Warsaw Ghetto investigators (37) and studies of patients with AIDS (38), is that humans do not survive once their BCM declines below approximately 60% of normal levels for young adults. Moreover, BCM declines steadily with age even in healthy, successfully ageing people (39, 40).

However, it is important to recognize that BCM can erode without a parallel loss of body weight. In fact, BCM can be lost in the face of increasing weight if there is a simultaneous increase in the mass of another compartment. For example, early in the course of congestive heart failure, cirrhosis or renal failure, an increase in extracellular fluid, resulting in increased weight (41–45), often masks BCM loss. Similarly, where ageing and rheumatoid arthritis are concerned (46, 47), an increase in fat mass often exceeds loss of BCM in absolute terms. Under these circumstances, dietary energy intake is generally normal while weight is stable or rising; weight loss and wasting occur later.

3.1.4 *Sarcopenia*

Sarcopenia—meaning literally a deficiency of flesh or muscle—develops even in healthy, successfully ageing adults and does not depend on the onset of disease. Sarcopenia's underlying mechanisms, which are probably diverse, have been reviewed elsewhere (48, 49). Its multifactorial etiology includes biological changes of ageing (loss of motor neurons, decrease in anabolic hormonal influences); disuse atrophy secondary to declining physical activities, which require high or rapid force output from muscle; and, in some cases, protein or energy undernutrition or catabolic disease processes such as congestive heart failure, rheumatoid arthritis, hyperthyroidism, Parkinson disease, and chronic infection or inflammation. In both healthy and frail older people, muscle fibre atrophy appears to be almost entirely limited to the Type II, or fast-twitch, fibres, as shown in the comparison of young and old cross-sectional fibre areas from muscle biopsy specimens of the *vastus lateralis*. Such selective atrophy, which can be produced in young individuals with experimental removal of gravity or muscle contraction, suggests a primary role in the etiology for muscle disuse.

3.1.5 **Fat mass**

Fat mass also changes, with an approximate doubling of body fat between 20 and 60 years of age, followed by progressive decline parallel to body mass index (BMI). Fat, which is the body's energy depot, has recently been recognized as playing a role in regulating energy intake and metabolism via leptin production (50–52). High fat mass is a risk factor for many diseases affecting older persons, including coronary heart disease, high blood pressure, diabetes, gallstones, osteoarthritis, and cancers of the breast and prostate (53). Increased obesity, especially obesity distributed predominantly in the abdominal (visceral) area, is associated with insulin resistance, which in turn causes diabetes and may also play a role in hypertension and hyperlipidaemia. The latter association may be a result of fat being a storehouse of fat-soluble carcinogens, or because fat cells produce low levels of estrogen, which may be important in postmenopausal women or for other unclear reasons. Assessment of fat mass and its distribution is thus important to understanding the health status and risk profile of older persons.

3.1.6 **Changes in bone**

Ageing is typically associated with a loss of bone and total body calcium. Women at all ages have lower total bone mass or total body calcium than men. Over a lifetime, women lose about 40% of their skeletal calcium, approximately one half in the first five years after menopause and the remainder at a slower rate thereafter. During the five years following menopause, it is impossible to prevent bone mineral loss with calcium supplementation alone. On the other hand, given the widely prevalent low calcium intakes (under 400 mg per day) seen in the USA, for example, later postmenopausal women benefit significantly—at the femoral neck, spine and radius—from calcium supplementation. In those subjects with intakes in the intermediate range of 400–650 mg, the effect of supplementation with calcium to the level of the 800 mg RDA is less striking. Some investigators have suggested that optimal calcium intake for a postmenopausal woman on a western diet is as high as 1400 mg per day. It is important to note that calcium needs are increased markedly by high dietary levels of sodium and protein, both of which increase urinary calcium excretion and thus result in more bone resorption if intake does not match output. A western diet, which is typically high in both sodium and protein, may thus contribute to the difficulty of maintaining bone mass in older persons and achieving calcium homeostasis.

Inadequate vitamin D intake

Inadequate vitamin D intake can also lead to bone loss and increased risk of osteoporosis. It has long been known in the Northern Hemisphere, for example, that serum levels of 25-hydroxyvitamin D—the best clinical index of vitamin D status—are higher in summer and autumn than in winter and spring. In addition to the general finding of seasonal variation in 25-hydroxyvitamin D, levels of this metabolite decline with age. Reduced levels of 25-hydroxyvitamin D in older persons result from declining intake, decreased sun exposure and, perhaps most importantly, less efficient skin synthesis of vitamin D.

Dawson-Hughes et al. (*54*) reported that 25-hydroxyvitamin D levels were lower in winter only among healthy postmenopausal women with daily vitamin D intakes under 220 IU. Those women with low vitamin D intakes had intact parathyroid hormone levels that were higher, although still within the normal range. Treatment of this population with a 400 IU vitamin D supplement prevented significant seasonal variation in either 25-hydroxyvitamin D or parathyroid hormone and, more importantly, reduced wintertime bone loss from the spine. During this vitamin D trial, both the placebo and supplemented groups had similar significant gains in bone density of the spine and whole body in the summer/autumn. Overall, there was a significant net benefit at the spine from vitamin D supplementation.

Those subjects exhibiting seasonal bone changes (increases in summer/autumn, decreases in winter/spring) also experience seasonal changes of similar magnitude in lean tissue mass. As indicated earlier, moderate changes in body composition can have a significant impact on level of function in older persons. Much is still to be learned about why bone, and lean and fat tissues, fluctuate with the seasons. Potential contributors to these circannual changes include seasonal differences in exercise, nutrition and blood levels of hormones that are known to affect the metabolism of these three tissue compartments.

Fractures

In Chapuy's (*55*) vitamin D and calcium study, fracture rates between controls and supplemented subjects began to diverge two months into the study, and the level of bone density increment was modest in the subset (1–3%) measured. This suggests that the result was due either to a reduction in falls or to a change in bone tensile strength rather than to an improvement in bone density, which was still far below the fracture threshold after supplementation. Similarly, in the Dawson-Hughes (*54*) calcium and vitamin D trial, fracture rates between groups diverged, early and progressively, despite a levelling off of bone density benefits after the first year of treatment.

In most cases hip fractures result from an injurious fall in persons with osteopenia. Prevention of hip fracture thus requires attention to both fall-related risk factors and bone density. Nutritional factors associated with traumatic hip fracture include protein-calorie malnutrition, alcohol abuse, osteomalaecia, low BMI, low muscle mass and strength, low levels of body fat, and low amounts of soft-tissue padding over the greater trochanteric region. For some of these factors, the association may be due to both increased risk of falling (e.g. muscle weakness from vitamin D deficiency, loss of balance from alcohol intoxication) and direct effects on skeletal integrity.

It is not known if adipose tissue is protective due to its shock-absorbing effect over the hip, to increased weight-bearing forces on bone over time due to adipose tissue mass, or to enhanced peripheral conversion of androgens to estrogens in women with more body fat. Once a hip fracture has occurred, there is evidence from a controlled clinical trial that rehabilitation is more successful if perioperative nutritional supplementation is begun immediately in hospital. More work is needed to identify gait and balance disorders associated with both vitamin D deficiency and protein-calorie malnutrition so that these factors are considered in the mainstream of both prevention and treatment of recurrent hip fracture in the elderly.

3.2 Changes in energy regulation with age

Energy intakes exceeding energy expenditure—described as positive energy balance—can explain the increase in body fat mass through middle age, although very little is known about the relative importance of overeating versus low energy expenditure. Conversely, negative energy balance is the primary cause of loss of body fat in old age. Since protein balance is closely linked to energy balance, this negative energy balance may also be the cause of loss of body protein in old age even when a protein-adequate diet is consumed. Thus, in addition to being a primary factor in changes in energy balance during the life cycle, age-associated alterations in energy regulation may also contribute to sarcopenia, which itself is linked to disability and frailty in old age.

3.2.1 *Low dietary energy intake*

Nationwide studies in the USA on weight and fat loss in old age suggest that low dietary energy intake is common among healthy older adults (56). Factors such as reduced sense of taste and smell, difficulties in chewing because of poor-fitting dentures or oral health problems, and difficulties in swallowing may also limit nutrient intake. Another factor may be depression, which is associated with weight gain in young adults but with weight loss in older persons (57). The diminished ability of older persons to control food intake, the so-called anorexia of ageing

(*58*), is also considered to be an important factor in energy regulation. Malabsorption and maldigestion are not characteristic of normal ageing since digestive and absorptive functions appear to be maintained up to age 100 in high-income countries (*59*). However, chronic intestinal infections and malnutrition can result in impaired functioning of the gastrointestinal tract with age for people in low-income countries.

While acknowledging the need for data on the possibility of alterations in energy requirements, Durnin (1990) suggested, on theoretical grounds, that current recommended dietary allowances might be expected to underestimate usual energy needs in older individuals (*60*).

The effects of age on energy requirements and control of food intake were investigated in 35 healthy sedentary men as a part of a larger investigation into metabolic responses to overeating and undereating (*61*). Subjects, who were encouraged to pursue their normal lifestyle and activities, kept a record of the type and duration of sports and other strenuous physical activities performed on each study day. As expected, the older men were significantly fatter and somewhat heavier than the younger men (*62*). The average daily duration of activities which the subjects themselves judged to be strenuous was similar in the two age groups, and it approximated the amount of strenuous activity anticipated in the current RDA for energy (*63*). However, the duration of truly strenuous activities (defined as those self-reported strenuous activities that had an expected energy expenditure of > 5 multiples of the resting energy expenditure) (*64*) was significantly reduced in the older group, which included such non-strenuous activities as walking in self-reports.

3.2.2 *Taste sensitivity and energy regulation*

Since taste sensitivity typically declines substantially with age (*65*), it is a potential factor contributing to changes in energy regulation associated with ageing. Approximately 25% of adults over age 65 have a reduced ability to detect one or more of the four basic tastes (sweet, sour, salty and bitter) at threshold concentrations (*66–68*) due to a reduction in the number and function of the tongue's taste papillae (*69*). In addition, fully 50% are unable to recognize blended foods in blind tests (*70*), which can be largely attributed to decrements in smell and taste in the older population (*71*). This is significant in view of the importance of smell and taste for determining overall sensory input and enjoyment from eating (*72*).

It is uncertain whether these alterations in taste sensitivity contribute to changes in energy regulation associated with ageing (*72*). Most people, including older adults (*73*), eat individual foods because they find them palatable. Thus, in theory, if reductions in taste sensitivity lead to reductions in perceived palatability, food intake could be adversely affected. However, such an association has not yet been demonstrated. Moreover, reports suggest that older individuals adapt to their reduced taste sensitivity and, for example, come to prefer foods with a lower salt concentration (74). In obvious contrast to this finding, Schiffman et al. (70) demonstrated increased enjoyment of meals spiked with flavours to compensate for reductions in taste sensitivity in older individuals, although investigators were unable to link greater enjoyment to increased intake. Changes in taste sensitivity undoubtedly occur with advancing age. Nevertheless, further studies are needed to understand better the effects of these changes on energy regulation.

3.3 Water metabolism and dehydration

Dehydration is a common, often readily preventable and potentially lethal problem among both institutionalized and community-dwelling older adults. In the USA, in 1991 more than 189 000 patients over age 65 were discharged from acute care hospitals with a primary diagnosis of dehydration (75). This translates into about 1.5% of community-dwelling older persons being hospitalized with dehydration each year (76). In community-dwelling older persons who developed progressive disability, dehydration was one of the most common diagnoses on admission to hospital (77). In 1991 the cost to Medicare of dehydration hospitalizations in the USA was over $US 1.1 billion (75).

3.3.1 *Etiology of dehydration in older persons*

In simple terms, older adults are at risk of dehydration due to reduced fluid intake and increased fluid loss (75). Even healthy older adults feel less thirst in response to water deprivation; this is evidenced both in a lower self-reported thirst score during dehydration and reduced intake of water after the dehydration period (78). In several studies, older subjects were not able to return to baseline plasma osmolality and sodium concentration despite free availability of water (78, 79). Fluid intake in young subjects, but not in older subjects, is modified by injection of naloxone, an opiate antagonist, suggesting that the opioid receptor system may be deficient in older adults and may contribute to the hypodypsia seen in older persons (80). In addition, with ageing there is a reduction in renal concentrating capacity in response to dehydration known as presbynephrosis, which contributes to the blunted ability of the elderly to defend against dehydration (79).

The defect in water homeostasis with ageing appears to be multifactorial but specific. Plasma renin activity and aldosterone secretion both diminish with age, as does the ability to respond to sodium deprivation with an appropriate increase in renin and aldosterone secretion (81). On the other hand, levels of plasma antidiuretic hormone (ADH) or arginine vasopressin (AVP) are elevated in older persons with dehydration compared to younger persons (78, 82), indicating that this portion of the volume and tonicity defence mechanism is not reduced with ageing. In fact, in contrast to their reduced ability to respond to dehydration, the ability of healthy older persons to respond to hypertonicity (induced by intravenous infusion of hypertonic saline) does not differ from that of younger adults (*83*).

These observations suggest that the defect in ageing relates more to the body's volume-sensing than to its tonicity-sensing mechanisms. However, until recently it has been difficult to distinguish between these two pathways because both dehydration and hypertonic saline infusion simultaneously alter plasma osmolality and extracellular fluid volume (*84*). To address this question, a recent study used head-out water immersion, which increases hydrostatic pressure outside the body and drives blood into the thoracic cavity, thus expanding central blood volume by about 700 ml and leading to increased cardiac filling pressure and heart volume without altering plasma osmolality (*84*). The increased central volume seems to activate cardiac stretch receptors, attenuating thirst and drinking; this effect is markedly diminished in healthy older subjects, despite a comparable, or greater, increase in central blood volume and atrial natriuretic peptide (*84*). This experiment suggests that a centrally mediated response to volume, but not to osmolality, is reduced with ageing.

The changes listed above seem to be physiologic since they occur in healthy older subjects in the absence of chronic diseases. However, many degenerative age-related diseases worsen the tendency towards dehydration in older persons. These include delirium, dementia, diuretic use, swallowing problems, laxative abuse, and problems with hand dexterity or ambulation. In addition, dehydration is a common complication of acute illness in older persons. For example, among Medicare beneficiaries in the USA hospitalized with dehydration, 28% had pneumonia or influenza, 25% had a urinary tract infection and 10% had gastro-enteritis (*76, 85*).

3.3.2 *Clinical evaluation*

Traditionally, dehydration has been classified by type according to water and sodium loss ratio. *Isotonic dehydration* indicates water and sodium loss comparable to that occurring during fasting, vomiting and diarrhoea. *Hypertonic dehydration* occurs when water loss exceeds sodium loss, and sodium levels rise above 145 mmol/l (or, according to some observers, 148 mmol/l), and serum osmolality rises above 300 mmol/kg. This is most commonly seen in older persons during fever and with a limited increase in oral fluid intake (*75*). *Hypotonic dehydration* occurs when sodium loss is greater than water loss, so that sodium falls below 135 mmol/l and osmolality is reduced to below 280 mmol/kg. Examples of this type of dehydration include diuretic excess and iatrogenic use of hyponatraemic intravenous fluids.

Unfortunately, recognizing dehydration still requires a modicum of clinical acumen; no single laboratory test is definitive. Weinberg and Minaker (*75*) suggest rapid and unintentional loss of > 3% of baseline body weight is a useful definition, but this approach is operational only if baseline weight is known and weight can be measured with sufficient accuracy. The variation in weight between scales is often greater than 3%, but healthy adults maintain their weight within this range over time (38). A history indicating risk factors for dehydration, e.g. fever, altered mental status and limited mobility, should alert the clinician to the possible presence of dehydration. Constipation is a common—and often the only—complaint in dehydrated older adults. In nursing-home residents, indication of declining urinary output may be helpful, but this is of limited value in incontinent patients.

Physical examination remains a crucial part of assessing hydration status. Unfortunately, signs of dehydration are often absent until the condition is far advanced. For example, age-related loss of subcutaneous tissue makes skin-tenting an unreliable sign in older persons, while dry mucus membranes may be present because of medications, breathing through the mouth or poorly fitting dentures. Orthostatic hypotension is usually a useful sign, but it may be absent if patients have cardiac conduction abnormalities, are fitted with a pacemaker or are taking β-blockers. In addition, false-positive orthostatic hypotension can be seen in a high proportion of normally hydrated older adults (86). Clinicians should use the constellation of these findings in the proper historical setting to accurately diagnose dehydration.

Laboratory tests that support the diagnosis can be obtained in most clinical situations. These include measuring blood urea nitrogen (BUN) and the BUN-to-creatinine ratio, serum osmolality, urine-specific gravity or osmolality, and perhaps plasma-specific gravity (75). These tests are also subject to false-positive and false-negative results and should be interpreted with caution. For example, an elevated BUN/creatinine ratio can occur as a result of gastrointestinal bleeding, obstructive uropathy or corticosteroid-induced muscle catabolism; serum osmolality can be increased as a result of hyperglycaemia, uraemia, hyperlipidaemia or ethanol ingestion; and urine-specific gravity and osmolality can be increased by glycosuria and may be falsely normal if renal disease causes isosthenuria. If serum osmolality is not available, it can be estimated using the following formula:

Osmolality (mOsm/kg) = serum sodium (mmol/l) + (glucose (mg/dl)/18) + (BUN (mg/dl)/2.8)

3.3.3 *Treating dehydration*

Although intravenous fluids are the obvious and rapid way to treat dehydration in an acute-care hospital, this may not be a feasible approach in other settings. Alternatives include oral fluids given by a caregiver with close observation of adequate intake; use of tube feeding with supplemental free water (since commercial formulas do not contain enough free water to replete someone who is dehydrated); and hypodermoclysis, the subcutaneous infusion of isotonic or hypotonic solution (87).

As a rule of thumb, adults require about 30 ml/kg of water per day (*75, 88*). However, because this level of intake may provide insufficient fluid to underweight adults, an alternative is to provide 100 ml/kg for the first 10 kg, 50 ml/kg for the next 10 kg and 15 ml/kg for the remaining weight (*88*). Even underweight adults should receive at least 1500 ml of fluid per day unless there is renal failure or another reason to restrict fluid intake. In hypernatraemic dehydration, the free water deficit (FWD) can be calculated using the following formula (*75*):

FWD (l) = weight (kg) x 0.45 – ([140/measured serum sodium] x weight (kg) x 0.45).

However, to be valid the baseline (i.e. normally hydrated) weight must be used in the formula, and this information may not always be available. In any case, rehydration of frail, older patients should be done under close supervision, with frequent monitoring of the clinical examination and laboratory tests to prevent both overhydration and inadequate rehydration.

3.4 **Immune function**

Considerable evidence indicates that ageing is associated with altered regulation of the immune system (*89*). Dysregulation of immune function contributes to the increased incidence of infectious, inflammatory and neoplastic diseases observed in older persons and to their prolonged post-illness recovery periods. The illness patterns in the elderly reflect both a deterioration of immune function and increased incidence of upper respiratory infections, shingles, tuberculosis and cancer. Moreover, prospective studies indicate that older persons with low delayed-type hypersensitivity skin test (DTH) responses have higher morbidity, are less self-sufficient, and have a higher incidence of post-operative complications and mortality compared with those with normal DTH responses (*90–92*).

There are two main types of immunity: innate or natural immunity, and acquired immunity (*93*). Innate immunity involves immune surveillance and killing mechanisms that do not require a previous encounter with a foreign substance by immune cells. Examples include phagocytosis by neutrophils and macrophages (M) and the tumoricidal and viricidal activities of natural killer (NK) cells. In contrast, acquired immunity necessitates an encounter with an antigen for the priming of a specific immune response. Acquired immunity involves M, T and B cells, and includes cell-mediated functions and humoral immunity or antibody production.

The dysregulation of immune function with ageing is well established (*94, 95*); it contributes to higher incidence of, and increased morbidity and mortality from, cancer and infectious autoimmune and neoplastic diseases (*91, 92*). A large part of the overall decline is made up of decreases in T cell-mediated function, including thymus involution and in vivo decreases in DTH response; the graft-versus-host reaction; resistance to tumours, viruses and parasites; T cell-dependent primary and secondary antibody responses; and the proportion of T cell subsets with naive cell surface markers (*93*). In addition, in vitro mitogen-stimulated lymphocyte proliferation, interleukin-2 (IL-2) production and responsiveness to IL-2 have been shown to decline with age. It appears that decreases and dysfunctions in cell function occur largely as a result of the decreased ability of ageing cells to receive and respond to cell signals (*97–101*). Some decline is also seen in humoral immune function, particularly in the loss of high-affinity cell surface receptors for antigens and cytokines.

Proliferation of B cells is fairly well maintained; however, old animals show impaired response to antigens that stimulate CD5+ B cells (foreign antigens). On the other hand, the ability of CD5+ B cells to respond to auto-antigens remains intact (*102*). Thus, while the ability to respond to foreign antigens declines with age, autoantibody formation increases with age, which may contribute to autoimmune disease (*103–105*). This dysregulated immune response is also observed in T cells in which production of Th1 cytokines is decreased, while production of Th2 cytokines is reported to increase with age (*106*). Furthermore, increased production of suppressive factors, e.g. prostaglandin (PG) E2 by M, has been reported to contribute to the dysregulation of T cell function (*107, 108*). However, there is no clear consensus on age-related changes in NK activity. Reviews on research in NK activity (*109, 110*) summarize reports of decrease, stasis and increase in NK activity with ageing. Differences in sample size, criteria used for including healthy older persons, age range and contamination by other cell types are possible contributing factors to these wide-ranging results (*111*).

Several macro- and micronutrients have been shown to play a regulatory role in immune system maintenance. Marginal and severe deficiencies of some of these nutrients are associated with impairments of T cell-mediated functions similar to those observed with ageing (*112*). Furthermore, supplementation with higher than the recommended dietary levels of some nutrients, e.g. vitamin E, has been shown to enhance immune response (*113*).

Several investigators have suggested that the nutritional status of older persons may be less than optimal, thereby contributing to immunological changes. Nutrient intake is often compromised in older persons due to chronic diseases as well as economic, psychosocial, physical and drug-related problems. Intakes below the RDA have been reported for zinc and vitamins E, C, and B6 (*114*). Supplementation at or above the RDA level for a single nutrient, or a mixture of nutrients, may thus prevent and/or delay the onset of age-related immunological defects.

Chandra & Puri (*115*) showed that nutritional supplementation of 30 malnourished men aged 70–84 years improved their antibody response to influenza vaccine. Lesourd et al. (*116*) studied the effect of protein-calorie undernutrition in three populations defined using the SENIEUR Protocol (*117*): *healthy young adults*

(20–50 years), *healthy older subjects* (mean age 79) and *healthy older subjects* (mean age 79) *with low nutritional status* (defined by a serum albumin level between 30 and 35 g/l). The authors noted that while certain indices of immune response (per cent CD3+ cells, mitogenic response, IL-2 production and antibody response to influenza vaccine) were lower in both groups of older persons compared with the young-adult group, other indices, e.g. per cent of CD4+ cells and DTH, were lower only in the undernourished older group compared with the young-adult group. Furthermore, in almost all indices examined, the age-related difference was more pronounced in the undernourished group. Lesourd et al. (*116*) also demonstrated that the magnitude of the decrease in nutritional status (determined by serum albumin levels) was important in determining the immune response in older persons, i.e. the lower the serum albumin levels, the lower the immune response. It is important to note that in these studies the low albumin level was not due to the presence of disease but was rather a reflection of low nutritional status.

These studies clearly demonstrate that undernutrition contributes to the decline of immune response with ageing. This is further supported by the observation that the immune response in undernourished older persons supplemented with 500 kcal$_{th}$/day[1] of a ready-to-use complete nutritional supplement was significantly higher than non-supplemented undernourished older people (*116*). However, it is not clear from these studies how much of the effect is due to protein-calorie undernutrition and how much is due to micronutrient deficiencies present under these conditions.

3.4.1 *Polyunsaturated fatty acids*
Certain types of fatty acids also have been shown to influence the immune response of older persons. Increasing intake of marine-derived *n*-3 polyunsaturated fatty acids (PUFA) was shown to decrease both the in vitro and in vivo indices of T cell-mediated function in healthy older persons (*118, 119*). This effect was specific to marine-derived *n*-3 PUFA and was not observed by increasing the intake of plant-derived *n*-6 PUFA (*119*). While the *n*-3 PUFA-induced decrease in T cell-mediated function would be considered an undesirable effect, higher intake does have the beneficial result of reducing the production of proinflammatory cytokines such as interleukin IL-1 and tumour necrosis factor (*118, 119*) as well as the production of eicosanoids such as prostaglandin (PG) E2 and leukotriene (LT) B4. Meydani et al. (*118*) showed that the *n*-3 PUFA-induced depression of T cell-mediated function was due to increased production of lipid peroxides, which can be prevented, at least in primates, by increasing vitamin E intake (*120*). Since high *n*-3 PUFA intake has been shown to reduce the risk of inflammatory coronary heart disease, further studies are needed to determine the appropriate tocopherol level needed to prevent

---

[1] 1000 kcal$_{th}$ is equivalent to 4.18 MJ.

the suppressive effect of fish oil on T cells while preserving the beneficial effect of reducing proinflammatory cytokines and eicosanoids.

3.4.2 *Vitamin B6*

Talbott et al. (*121*) examined the effect on lymphocyte response in a group of eleven healthy individuals over 65 years of age of supplementation for two months with 50 mg/day of vitamin B6. The vitamin B6-supplemented group showed a significant increase in lymphocyte proliferation in response to T and B cell mitogens relative to a placebo control group of four older subjects. Percentages of helper (but not suppresser/cytotoxic) T cells increased significantly in the pyridoxine-treated subjects. The supplementation was more effective in those subjects with the lowest initial plasma pyridoxal phosphate levels, indicating that higher than RDA levels of B6 might be needed to achieve optimal immune responsiveness in older persons. This is supported by the study by Meydani et al. (*122*) who, using a B6 depletion–repletion protocol, showed that IL-2 production and mitogenic response to T and B cell mitogens by peripheral blood mononuclear cells of older subjects are influenced by changes in dietary vitamin B6 levels. In this study, biochemical measures of vitamin B6 status returned to normal at dosages of 1.90–1.96 mg/day. At this dosage, however, lymphopenia secondary to vitamin B6 depletion was not corrected. Furthermore, IL-2 production and mitogenic response in at least half the subjects were still below baseline level, indicating that either a longer period of supplementation at this level or a higher level of vitamin B6 are needed to normalize immune response.

3.4.3 *Vitamin E*

In a double-blind placebo-controlled study, Meydani et al. (*123*) showed that supplementation of healthy older subjects (over age 60) with vitamin E (800 IU/day of dl-α-tocopheryl acetate) for 30 days significantly improved DTH response, lymphocyte proliferative response to the T cell mitogen concanavalin A (Con A), and Con A-stimulated IL-2 production. To determine the optimal level of vitamin E, Meydani et al. (*124*) supplemented healthy older subjects (over age 65) with either a placebo, 60 mg/day, 200 mg/day or 800 mg/day of dl-α-tocopheryl acetate for 235 days using a double-blind randomized design. All three vitamin E doses significantly enhanced DTH; however, subjects consuming 200 mg/day of vitamin E had the highest per cent increase in DTH. The median per cent change in DTH in the subjects supplemented with 200 mg/day vitamin E (65%) was significantly higher than that of the placebo group (17%). Although the median per cent change in the groups supplemented with 60 and 800 mg/day vitamin E (41% and 49%, respectively) was similar to the 65% change observed in the 200 mg/day group, these changes did not reach statistical significance compared with those of the placebo group.

There was no significant effect of supplementation with 60 mg/day of vitamin E on response to hepatitis B or tetanus and diphtheria vaccines. However, a significant increase in antibody response to hepatitis B was observed in subjects consuming 200 or 800 mg/day of vitamin E. Subjects consuming 200 mg/day also had a significant increase in antibody response to tetanus toxoid vaccine. Vitamin E supplementation had no effect on either the level of two autoantibodies, anti-DNA and anti-thyroglobulin, or the ability of neutrophils to kill *Candida albicans*. These data suggest that while supplementation with 60 mg/day of vitamin E might enhance DTH, it is inadequate to cause a significant increase in antibody titre against hepatitis B or tetanus toxoid. Supplementation with 200 mg/day of vitamin E, however, caused a significant increase in DTH and antibody response, and the magnitude of response for both indices was higher than those observed in the two other vitamin E groups.

It was thus concluded that 200 mg/day represents the optimal level of vitamin E for enhancing the immune response of older persons. The observation that the optimal response was detected in the 200 mg/day group suggests that there may be a threshold level for the immunostimulatory effect of vitamin E. Interestingly, vitamin E-supplemented subjects had a 30% lower incidence of self-reported infections, indicating that the immunostimulatory effect of vitamin E might have clinical significance for older persons.

This possibility is supported by studies conducted in laboratory animals. Hayek et al. (*125*) fed young and old mice either 30 or 500 parts per million (ppm) vitamin E for 8 weeks, at which time they were infected with influenza virus. Old mice fed 30 ppm of vitamin E had higher viral titres than young mice fed the same way. Influenza lung viral titres were lower in old mice fed 500 ppm vitamin E compared with the age-matched mice fed 30 ppm vitamin E. In a subsequent study, Han et al. (*126*) showed that the preventive effect of vitamin E was not observed following supplementation with other antioxidant compounds such as glutathione, melatonin or strawberry extract. Furthermore, vitamin E prevented the weight loss associated with influenza infection, while other dietary antioxidant treatments had no effect on weight loss.

The immunostimulatory effect of vitamin E on T cell function was not observed with another antioxidant, β-carotene. Santos et al. (*127*) showed that neither short-term, high-dose (90 mg/day for 3 weeks) nor long-term, moderate-dose (50 mg every 2 days for 12 years) supplementation with β-carotene had a significant effect on in vitro or in vivo indices of T cell-mediated function. However, long-term β-carotene supplementation did increase natural killer cell activity in older people (*128*).

No adverse effects due to vitamin E supplementation were observed on the immune indices tested. Recently, the safety in older subjects of four months of supplementation with 60, 200 and 800 IU/day of dl-α-tocopheryl acetate was assessed in terms of general health, nutrient status, liver enzyme function, thyroid hormones, creatine levels, serum autoantibodies, killing of *Candida albicans* by neutrophils, and bleeding time. Supplementation with vitamin E at these levels and for this period had no adverse effects on these parameters (*129*).

3.4.4 *Selenium*

Selenium has been shown to be an essential nutrient for maintaining immune response. Recent animal studies indicate that selenium supplementation might improve immune response in older persons. Kiremidjian-Schumacher & Roy (*130*) showed that 24-month-old mice supplemented with 2.0 ppm selenium for eight weeks had higher mitogenic response to PHA (phytohaemagglutinin) and cytolytic T lymphocyte activity against malignant cells than non-supplemented mice. This effect was not due to increases in IL-1, IL-2 or INF (interferon) gamma-production, but rather to selenium's ability to enhance the expression of (p55) and/or β (p70/75) subunits of the IL-2 R on the surface of activated cells.

A six-month, double-blind, placebo-controlled trial of selenium supplementation (100 µg/day as selenium-enriched yeast) in institutionalized older persons (mean age 78 years, $n=22$) showed significantly greater lymphocyte proliferation in response to pokeweed mitogen (*131*). This increase in proliferative response was limited to B cells and was not exhibited in proliferative responses to T cell mitogens PHA or OKT3. No significant correlations between plasma selenium levels and lympho-proliferative responses were established, although it is interesting to note that the greatest increases in B cell proliferation occurred in subjects who had the lowest plasma selenium levels at baseline. Although the authors concluded on this basis that selenium supplementation enhances immune response in older persons, this is not supported by the data presented. As mentioned above, the main age-related difference occurs in T cell-mediated function. Since selenium supplementation in this study did not improve mitogenic response to T cell mitogens, selenium supplementation was not effective in changing the age-associated defect in T cells.

3.4.5 *Zinc*

Several investigators have evaluated, with conflicting results, the effect of zinc supplementation on the immune response of older subjects (*132*). A recent study (*133*) utilized a double-blind placebo-controlled design where subjects were randomly assigned to a placebo group or groups receiving 15 or 100 mg/day of zinc sulphate. All groups received a multivitamin/mineral supplement containing 20 to 300% RDA of several vitamins and minerals known to be required for optimal immune response. These included vitamin E (250% of RDA), folate (100% of RDA), pyridoxine (150% of RDA), vitamin A (138% of RDA), selenium (20% of RDA) and iron (270% of RDA). Except for a transient improvement in NK cell activity, no significant improvement in indices of the immune response (mitogenic response and DTH) was observed due to zinc supplementation. However, all three groups showed improvement in DTH, with the placebo group (which also received multivitamin/mineral supplements) showing the largest increase (P< 0.01) compared to the groups receiving zinc supplements. The authors speculated that the improvement observed in the placebo group was due to the multivitamin/ mineral supplement and not to a boosting effect caused by repeated administration of DTH (multi-test cell-mediated immunity, which does not have a boosting effect when used in time intervals of more than one month, was used in this study).

3.4.6 *Multivitamin/mineral supplementation*

This finding was later confirmed in studies by Bogden et al. (*134*) and Chandra et al. (*135*). Bogden et al. (134) showed that one year of supplementation with a daily micronutrient formulation containing 1–2 times the RDA level of several micronutrients significantly improved DTH response. Chandra et al. (*135*) investigated the effect of year-long supplementation with a multivitamin/mineral supplement on immune response and frequency of infectious diseases in healthy men and women over 65 years of age. With the exception of vitamin E and β-carotene, the supplement contained 0.5–2 times the RDA for nutrients while the placebo capsules contained 200 mg of calcium and 100 mg of magnesium. Nutrient blood levels were compared to normal reference standards (NRS) established by analysing fasting blood from 38 to 141 healthy subjects (age 66–68 years) living in St John's, Newfoundland. These subjects were followed for one to three years after nutrient analysis, and values from those who remained healthy were used to develop the NRS. For the supplementation trial, subjects were considered deficient in a particular nutrient if their nutrient values fell below the 95% confidence limits of these NRS values.

The placebo and supplemented groups had a similar prevalence of nutrient deficiency which, compared to NRS values, varied from 2.1% for selenium to 18.7% for vitamin C. While there was no significant difference in deficiency prevalence between the two groups at baseline, the supplemented group tended to have a higher prevalence of nutrient deficiency. No change in prevalence of nutrient deficiency was observed in the placebo group during the 12-month treatment period. However, a significant reduction was observed in the prevalence of deficiency, in the supplemented group, in vitamin A, β-carotene, vitamin B6, vitamin C, iron and zinc.

Significant improvements in several of the immunological tests were observed only in the supplemented group. No difference was observed in per cent of lymphocytes; however, a significant increase was observed in per cent of T cells (CD3+), helper T cells (CD4+) and NK cells. Mitogenic response to T cell mitogen PHA, IL-2 production and NK cell cytotoxicity were significantly improved in the supplemented group. Moreover, antibody response to influenza vaccine was higher in the supplemented group compared to the placebo group.

It is not clear which component of the supplement used by Bogden & Chandra resulted in the observed improvements. Several nutrients contained in the mixture—vitamins C, E and B6, β-carotene, selenium and zinc—are needed for normal immune response. Supplementation of older persons with higher than RDA levels of some of these nutrients—vitamins E and B6 separately, a combination of antioxidant nutrients (*136*), or a combination of antioxidants and B vitamins (*137*)—has been shown to improve this group's immune response. The contributions of individual supplement components could have been more easily determined if correlations between changes in immunological indices and changes in blood levels of specific nutrients had been reported. A subsequent study by Pike & Chandra (*138*), using the same supplement in an apparently healthier group of older subjects with fewer nutritional deficiencies, found no improvement in mitogenic response to T cell mitogens. The reason for this discrepancy is not clear, but it may be due to differences in health status and the prevalence of nutrient deficiencies in the two study populations.

Numerous studies have demonstrated that significant improvement in the immune response of healthy older persons can be achieved by nutrient supplementation, although the clinical significance of nutrient-induced immunological changes has been questioned. However, Chandra (*135*) found that immunological improvements following nutrient supplementation were associated with decreased frequency of infection-related illnesses. Furthermore, antibiotics were used for fewer days to treat infections in the supplemented group.

Meydani et al. (*124*) also reported a trend towards lower incidence of infectious disease in older subjects who were supplemented with vitamin E compared with a placebo group. Vitamin E supplementation (*125, 126*) has also been shown to reduce lung viral titres following influenza infection. The evidence thus far suggests that improved immune response following nutrient intervention might have clinical significance for this age group. However, further studies are needed to confirm these findings.

3.5 **Neurological and cognitive function**

Mental impairment and dementia as a result of chronic degenerative brain disease have a particularly severe impact on autonomy and independence. Indeed, the age-associated increase in mental impairment leading to dementia is probably the most serious threat to ageing populations. The prospect of postponing, or preventing altogether, the onset of disability due to cognitive impairment is thus of central importance to public health policy.

The clinically defined syndrome of dementia is most often caused by Alzheimer disease, followed by vascular dementia and, less frequently, by other more recently defined neurodegenerative disorders. To this latter group belong dementia with Lewy bodies (*139*), frontotemporal dementia (*140*) and dementia with Parkinson disease. Recent epidemiological research has established cerebrovascular disease's close links to Alzheimer disease with far-reaching implications for prevention (*141, 142*).

Depression, which is a very common symptom of these illnesses and is the most important mood disorder in older persons, is the functional answer to a wide variety of contributing factors (*143*). However, because depression also results from an imbalance of neurotransmitters, it is useful to distinguish between depression as a first manifestation of dementing disorders, e.g. Alzheimer disease, or true depressive states without the background of a defined structural disorder (*144*).

It is generally accepted that dementing illnesses and depression have a strong genetic background. Nevertheless, since the genetic susceptibility to a certain disease is strongly influenced by environmental factors, nutrients can have either a disease-accelerating or protective effect. For example, independently of genetic predisposition, certain nutrients or toxic substances can directly affect brain development (alcohol, folic-acid deficiency) or brain function (alcohol, vitamin B1 and B12 deficiencies). Mental symptoms such as cognitive impairment, emotional irritability or other neurological signs are well known in case of vitamin deficiencies.

3.5.1 *Effect of nutrients on brain function*

Conceptually, it is useful to distinguish between probable direct effects on cells of the central nervous system and effects influencing circulation—and hence the nutrient and oxygen supply—of brain tissue. Nutrition can have an impact on brain function by impairing energy supply; affecting neurotransmitter synthesis and intermediary metabolism; enhancing, or protecting from, oxidative stress; and influencing cytokines and other signalling molecules.

Impact of vascular disease

Diet is closely linked to vascular disease. Thus, long-standing hypertension and factors contributing to hypertension (e.g. obesity, high salt intake) and factors contributing to vascular disease (e.g. hyperlipidaemia, elevated homocysteine levels, diabetes mellitus, smoking) may already play an important role during childhood and have consequences in old age.

Large geographical variations clearly relate atherosclerosis of coronary and brain vessels to environmental factors. The impressive decline in stroke and cardiovascular disease (*145*) over the last three decades is in part related to active treatment of risk factors; but it is probably linked even more to improved nutrition, particularly the intake of water-soluble vitamins B and C. The striking fourfold higher stroke mortality (Figure 2) in subjects having simultaneously low plasma concentrations of vitamin C and carotene demonstrates that concentrations already at plasma levels in the low-normal range increase the risk for vascular diseases (*146*). It is now well recognized that high cardiovascular risk correlates with high stroke risk and thus with vascular dementia. In a study by Gale et al. (*147*) stroke was associated with low vitamin C intake and cognitive impairment was associated with stroke. This demonstrates the close relationship between stroke and vascular dementia, which also share common risk factors such as hypertension, smoking, diabetes mellitus, atrial fibrillation and, to a lesser extent, hyperlipidaemia (*141, 148, 149*). Homocysteine levels might be important, linking levels of folic acid, and vitamins B6 and B12, with vascular dementia (*150, 151*).

An interesting new aspect of low energy (glucose) supply is that it may lead to glutamate toxicity in vulnerable brain regions. Astrocytes clear glutamate from the synaptic cleft. Low glucose supply or impaired intermediary metabolism, e.g. due to lack of vitamin B1 or antioxidants, may impair glutamate uptake and expose neurons to exitoxicity (*152*).

Figure 2. **Combined low plasma levels of ß-carotene and vitamin C associated with significant increased risk for stroke**[a]

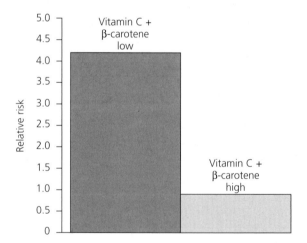

[a] *Adapted from reference 146 with the permission of the publisher.*

Neurotransmitter synthesis

Neurotransmitters are synthesized endogenously from precursors ingested as nutrients. Wurtman (153) demonstrated the competing effect of different amino acids, and hence the impact of transmitter precursors on uptake by the brain. In the fasting state and with high protein intake, large neutral amino acids compete for the tryptophan carrier, which leads to diminished serotonine synthesis. On the other hand, glucose intake raises insulin concentration, which in turn increases the uptake of large neutral amino acids in muscle and consequently enhances entry of tryptophan in the brain. Tryptophan depletion can induce a relapse in depressive patients (*154*).

Evidence supporting an association between folate deficiency and depressive symptoms was already reported in 1962 (*155*). One important step involving folate is the participation of tetra-hydro-biopterin (BH4) as a co-factor in the hydroxy-lation of phenylalanine and tryptophan, the precursors of dopamine, norepinefrine and serotonine. Thus, tissue concentration of folic acid and vitamin B12 may change independently of the effect on homocysteine, which may be a vascular toxin or possibly neurotoxic.

Cognitive function

A number of earlier studies reported better performance in cognitive tests in subjects with higher plasma levels or intake of a variety of vitamins. Both Goodwin et al. and Chome et al. found an association between micronutrient intake and cognitive performance (*156, 157*). In another study, Wahlin et al. observed better cognitive function in subjects with vitamin B12 levels above 200 pmol/l compared to lower levels (*158*). The authors conclude that subjects with intakes or plasma levels at the lower end perform less well compared to subjects with normal levels; that normal levels are sufficient for normal cognitive function; and that subnormal levels may be associated with cognitive impairment. These studies demonstrate a rapid and close interplay of nutrition, mood and behaviour, implying that intake of a wide variety of foods, and possibly supplements, is necessary to optimize brain function in older persons.

Since brain ageing is associated with oxidative stress, antioxidants are of particular interest. In the prospective Basel Study, which focused on cognitive changes during ageing (*159*), participants underwent a complete plasma vitamin analysis in 1971–1973 (*160*). In 1993, 452 participants aged 65 or older took part in further tests involving correlations between biological parameters and memory function. It is noteworthy that neither smoking nor blood pressure was predictive of better memory performance, but that subjects with high plasma vitamin C and β-carotene, even measured 20 years earlier, performed better. One concern in this kind of study is that higher educational and socioeconomic status concurrent with better micronutrient intake might lead to better memory performance. However, as Figure 3 (*159*) shows, the relationship is maintained even when different educational levels are reviewed.

The Basel Study's findings are supported by the Rotterdam Study (*161*) where low intake of β-carotene (< 0.9 mg/day) was associated with significantly poorer cognitive performance when compared to subjects with an intake of > 2.1 mg/day. The SENECA-EURONUT Investigation (*162*) analysed European subjects born

Figure 3. **Effects of age (young-old, old-old), education (primary, secondary, university), and plasma level of ascorbic acid (high, low) on performance in the WAIS-R vocabulary test[a]**

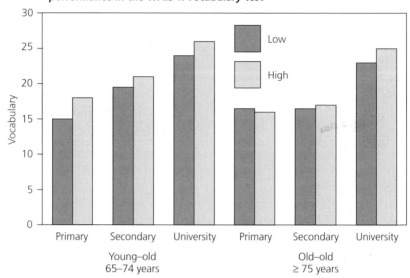

[a] *Reproduced from reference 159 with the permission of the publisher.*

between 1911 and 1914. It is noteworthy that concentrations of plasma carotene, vitamin C and α-tocopherol correlated with the Mini-Mental Status Examination, a cognitive function screening method for detecting dementing disorders. Of particular interest in this connection is the observation by de Rijk et al. (*163*) who suggest that a high intake of dietary vitamin E may protect against the occurrence of Parkinson disease.

Taken together, these data strongly suggest that as ageing continues, carotene and carotenoids, ascorbic acid and α-tocopherol influence brain function. In contrast to cardiovascular disease, there is no clear evidence suggesting additional benefits from intakes above RDAs. Primary preventive intervention trials showing a benefit in terms of delaying cognitive decline over time are not yet available. On theoretical grounds, a slowing of deterioration might be expected, but this is rather difficult to demonstrate in the absence of overt degenerative brain disease.

3.5.2 *Prevention and treatment of degenerative brain disease*

A review of the literature results in only a very limited number of studies investigating the effect of high doses of vitamins in primary degenerative dementias. A preliminary finding in one study of a favourable effect of very high thiamine dosages (3–8 g/day) in Alzheimer disease patients was not followed up with further investigation (*164*). The identification of free radical involvement in Parkinson disease formed the rationale for the study by Fahn et al. (*165, 166*) who evaluated the effect of high doses of vitamin E and ascorbic acid and reported that intake of 1800 IU of vitamin E and ascorbate delayed the necessity of dopa substitution by 2.4 years. However, this work has not yet been confirmed. In a longer follow-up study, no effect of α-tocopherol was seen when given in this high amount. In addition, the study did not clarify whether vitamin E in such amounts acts as an antioxidant only, or whether effects on microcirculation, or even pro-oxidant accents, could be important.

A recent study in patients with mild to moderate Alzheimer disease, (*167*) once again treated with 1800 IU α-tocopherol, found a significant slowing in deterioration of mental function compared to untreated controls, thus permitting a delay in institutionalization. The therapeutic effect was comparable to the impact of selegilin therapy alone. Interestingly, the combination of selegilin and α-tocopherol did not increase treatment effectiveness. The same caveats apply for this study as in the case of Parkinson disease. In addition, the high dose of vitamin E was not accompanied by an increased intake of ascorbic acid. Nevertheless, the pathophysiological rationale of antioxidants and B vitamins in chronic degenerative brain disease has opened new preventive and therapeutic possibilities for reducing and delaying age-associated mental decline. It may well be that vitamins will eventually be shown to contribute substantially to maintaining autonomy in old age.

3.5.3 *Zinc's role in dementia*

The Basel Study demonstrated an unfavourable effect on cognition of high iron concentration, thus supporting the oxidative stress hypothesis (*159*). The role of zinc, which is known to be diminished in the Alzheimer-diseased brain, is also of interest. Up to 15% of brain zinc is contained in synaptic vesicles (*168*), and the highest concentration is found in the hippocampus. The depletion observed in the Alzheimer-diseased brain may result from loss of synapses and neurones. Zinc enhances the formation of β-amyloid aggregation; thus, in the process of the degenerative disease, zinc may even accelerate the formation of neuritic plaques. Astrocytes play an important role in zinc metabolism; they contain high amounts of glutathione and glutathione disulphide, which are able to release zinc. Oxidative stress induces an increase in free zinc, which is involved in many enzyme actions that may be important in a wide variety of neurodegenerative disorders. Given the subsequent importance of zinc, the very commonly observed low levels of zinc in geriatric patients with dementia are difficult to interpret.

3.5.4 *Nutrients, cognitive function and mood*

Nutrients can affect cognitive function, mood and behaviour in older persons in several ways. Stroke and related disorders contribute significantly to disability in old age. The intake of protective micronutrients can lower the risk of stroke and related disorders by keeping the vascular system functioning adequately. It is likely that bioactive non-nutrients also play an underestimated role in supporting vascular function. Foods with high antioxidant properties can also protect against the damage caused by free radicals, a significant cause of brain ageing and loss of cognitive function. However, older persons are often unable to maintain a varied enough diet to obtain an appropriate amount of the necessary micronutrients. Supplements or food fortification may thus be necessary in at-risk populations.

4. **Impact of physical activity**

The age-associated loss of muscle mass called sarcopenia (*169*) is a direct cause of age-related decrease in muscle strength. Several teams have examined this issue. For example, Frontera et al. (*34*) studied muscle strength and mass in 200 healthy 45–78-year-old men and women and concluded that muscle mass (and not function) is the major determinant of the age and sex-related differences in strength. This relationship was independent of muscle location (upper versus lower extremities) and function (extension versus flexion). Reduced muscle strength in older persons is a major cause of their increased disability prevalence. With advancing age and the extremely low activity levels seen in the very old, muscle strength and power become critical aspects of walking ability (*170*). The high prevalence of falls among institutionalized older persons may well be a consequence of their reduced muscle strength.

4.1 **Impact of endurance training**

To what extent are these changes inevitable consequences of ageing? Data examining young and middle-aged endurance-trained men demonstrate that body fat stores and maximal aerobic capacity were not related to age, but rather to the total number of hours the men were exercising per week (*171*). Even among sedentary individuals, energy spent in daily activities explains more than 75% of the variability in body fat among young and older men (*172*). These data and the results of other investigations indicate that levels of physical activity are important in determining energy expenditure and, ultimately, body-fat accumulation. However, cross-sectional data from Klitgaard et al. indicate that older endurance athletes (runners and swimmers) display fat-free mass and muscle strength similar to that seen in sedentary aged-matched controls, suggesting that endurance exercise alone may not prevent sarcopenia (*173, 174*).

4.2 **Impact of aerobic exercise**

Aerobic exercise has long been an important recommendation for the prevention and treatment of many of the chronic diseases typically associated with old age. These include NIDDM and impaired glucose tolerance, hypertension, heart disease and osteoporosis. Regularly performed aerobic exercise increases VO2max (the maximum capacity to take in and use oxygen during exercise) and insulin action.

Meredith et al. (*175*) examined the responses of initially sedentary young (age 20–30) and older (age 60–70) men and women to three months of aerobic conditioning (70% of maximal heart rate, 45 minutes/day, three days per week). Absolute gains in aerobic capacity were found to be similar between the two age groups, although the mechanism for adaptation to regular submaximal exercise appears to be different.

Muscle biopsies taken before and after training showed a more than twofold increase in oxidative capacity of the muscles of the older subjects, while improvements in the muscles of the younger subjects were smaller. In addition, skeletal muscle glycogen stores in the older subjects—significantly lower initially than those of the younger men and women—increased significantly. The degree to which older persons demonstrate increases in maximal cardiac output in response to endurance training is still largely unanswered. Seals et al. (*176*) found no increases after one year of endurance training. In contrast, more recently Spina et al. (*177*) observed that older men increased maximal cardiac output, while healthy older women demonstrated no change in response to endurance exercise. If accurate, these sex-related cardiovascular differences may explain the lack of response in maximal cardiac output when older men and women are included in the same study population.

4.2.1 *Changes in glucose tolerance*

Exercise also has the potential to improve carbohydrate metabolism, which is frequently impaired in older individuals. The two-hour plasma glucose level during an oral glucose tolerance test increases by an average of 5.3 mg/dl per decade, and fasting plasma glucose increases by an average of 1 mg/dl per decade (*178*). The NHANES II study demonstrated a progressive increase of about 0.4 mM/decade of life in mean plasma glucose value two hours after a 75 g oral glucose tolerance test (*n*=1678 men and 1892 women) (*179*). Shimokata et al. (*180*) examined glucose tolerance in community-dwelling men and women ranging between age 17 and 92. By assessing fitness and obesity levels, patterns of body-fat distribution and activity in an attempt to examine the independent effect of age on glucose tolerance, investigators found no significant differences between the young and middle-aged groups. However, the older groups had significantly higher glucose and insulin values (following a glucose challenge) than the younger or middle-aged groups. The study's major finding—considered both unique and unexplained—was that, whereas the decline in glucose tolerance from the early-adult to the middle-age years is entirely accounted for by secondary influences (fat and fitness), the decline from mid-life to old age still is also influenced by chronological age.

However, it is important to note that anthropometric determination of body fat becomes increasingly less accurate with advancing age while it fails to reflect the intra-abdominal and intramuscular accumulation of fat that occurs with ageing

(*181*). The results of this study may in fact be due more to underestimating true body fat levels than to age per se. Age-associated changes in glucose tolerance can result in NIDDM and a broad array of associated abnormalities. Recently, in a large population of older men and women (over 55), serum glucose and fructosamine levels were seen to be higher in subjects with retinopathy compared with those without; and within the groups with retinopathy, serum glucose was significantly associated with number of haemorrhages (*182*). These relationships were independent of body composition, abdominal obesity or the presence of NIDDM.

The relationship between ageing, body composition, activity and glucose tolerance was also examined in 270 female and 462 male factory workers aged 22–73, none of whom was retired (*183*). Plasma glucose levels, both fasting and after a glucose load, increased with age, but the correlation between age and total integrated glucose response following a glucose load was weak; in women, only 3% of the variance could be attributed to age. When activity levels and drug use were factored in, age accounted for only 1% of the variance in women and 6.25% in men.

4.2.2 *Exercise in the treatment of glucose intolerance and NIDDM*

The significant effects that aerobic exercise has on skeletal muscle may help to explain its importance in the treatment of glucose intolerance and NIDDM. Seals et al. (*184*) found that a high-intensity training programme resulted in greater improvements in the insulin response to an oral glucose load compared to lower intensity aerobic exercise. However, subjects began the study with normal glucose tolerance. Kirwan et al. (*185*) found that 9 months (4 days/week) of endurance training at 80% of the maximal heart rate resulted in reduced glucose-stimulated insulin levels; however, no comparison was made to a lower intensity exercise group. Hughes et al. (*186*) demonstrated that regularly performed aerobic exercise without weight loss resulted in improved glucose tolerance, rate of insulin-stimulated glucose disposal and increased skeletal muscle GLUT-4 (the glucose-transporter protein in skeletal muscle) levels in older glucose-intolerant subjects. In this investigation, a moderate-intensity aerobic exercise programme was compared to a higher-intensity programme (50% versus 75% of maximal heart-rate reserve, 55 minutes/day 4 days/week for 12 weeks). No differences were seen in glucose tolerance between the moderate and higher intensity aerobic exercise, insulin sensitivity or muscle GLUT-4 levels. This appears to indicate that a moderate aerobic exercise programme should be recommended for older men or women who have NIDDM or are at risk of developing it.

Endurance training and dietary modifications are generally recommended as primary treatment for the non-insulin-dependent diabetic. Cross-sectional analysis of dietary intake supports the hypothesis that a low carbohydrate/high fat diet is associated with the onset of NIDDM (*187*). However, this evidence is not supported by prospective studies where dietary habits have been related to the development of NIDDM (*188, 189*). The effects of a high carbohydrate diet on glucose tolerance have been equivocal (*190, 191*). Hughes et al. (*192*) compared the effects of a high carbohydrate (60% carbohydrate and 20% fat)/high fibre (25 g dietary fibre/1000 kcal$_{th}$) diet with, and without, three months of high-intensity endurance exercise (75% maximal heart rate reserve, 50 minutes/day, four days/week) in older glucose-intolerant men and women. Subjects were fed all their food on a metabolic ward during the three-month study and were not allowed to lose weight. Investigators observed no improvement in glucose tolerance or insulin-stimulated glucose uptake in either the diet or the diet-plus-exercise group.

The exercise-plus-high-carbohydrate-diet group demonstrated a significant increase in skeletal muscle glycogen content, and muscle glycogen stores were considered saturated at the end of training. Since the primary site of glucose disposal is skeletal muscle glycogen stores, the extremely high muscle glycogen content associated with exercise and a high carbohydrate diet probably limited the rate of glucose disposal. When combined with exercise and a weight-maintenance diet, a high carbohydrate diet thus had a counter-regulatory effect. Recently, Schaefer et al. (*193*) demonstrated that older subjects lost weight consuming an ad libitum high-carbohydrate diet.

There appears to be no attenuation of the response of older men and women to regularly performed aerobic exercise when compared to that observed in younger subjects. Increased fitness levels are associated with reduced mortality and increased life expectancy, in addition to helping to prevent NIDDM (*194*) in subjects who are at the greatest risk of developing this disease. Regularly performed aerobic exercise is thus an important way for older people to improve their glucose tolerance.

Aerobic exercise is generally prescribed as an important adjunct to a weight-loss programme since it has been demonstrated that the two together increase insulin action to a greater extent than weight loss alone through dietary restriction. For example, in a study by Bogardus et al. (*195*), while diet therapy alone improved glucose tolerance mainly by reducing basal endogenous glucose production and enhancing hepatic sensitivity to insulin, aerobic exercise increased carbohydrate storage rates. However, aerobic exercise (as opposed to resistance training) combined with a hypocaloric diet have been shown to result in a greater reduction in resting metabolic rate (RMR) than that achieved by diet therapy alone (*196*). Heymsfield et al. (*197*) found that aerobic exercise combined with caloric restriction did not preserve fat-free mass and did not further accelerate weight loss when compared with diet therapy. The lack of impact of aerobic exercise may have been due to a greater decrease in RMR in the exercising group.

In perhaps the most comprehensive study of its kind, Goran & Poehlman (*198*) examined components of energy metabolism in older men and women engaged in regular endurance training. They found that endurance training did not increase total daily energy expenditure owing to a compensatory decline in physical activity during the remainder of the day. Thus, when older subjects participated in a regular walking program, they rested more and activities other than walking decreased, with the result that 24-hour calorie expenditure was unchanged. Nevertheless, older individuals who have participated in endurance exercise for most of their lives have been shown to have a higher RMR and total daily energy expenditure than age-matched sedentary controls (*199*). Ballor et al. (*200*) compared the effects of resistance training to that of diet restriction alone in obese women. They found that resistance exercise training resulted in increased strength and gains in muscle size as well as a preservation of fat-free mass during weight loss. These results are similar to those of Pavlou et al. (*201*) who used both aerobic and resistance training as an adjunct to a weight-loss programme for obese men.

4.3 Strength training to reduce loss of muscle mass

While endurance exercise has been the more traditional means of increasing cardiovascular fitness, the American College of Sports Medicine recommends strength or resistance training as an important component of an overall fitness programme. This is particularly important in older persons for whom loss of muscle mass and weakness are prominent features.

Strength conditioning, or progressive resistance training, is generally defined as training where the resistance against which a muscle generates force is progressively increased over time. Progressive resistance training involves a few contractions against a heavy load. The metabolic and morphological adaptations resulting from resistance and endurance exercise are quite different. Muscle strength has been shown to increase in response to training between 60 and 100% of the one repetition maximum (1RM), which is the maximum amount of weight that can be lifted with one contraction. Strength conditioning results in an increase in muscle size, which is largely the result of increased contractile proteins. The ways in which mechanical events stimulate an increase in ribonucleic acid (RNA) synthesis and subsequent protein synthesis are not well understood. Lifting weight requires a muscle to shorten as it produces force, and this is called a concentric contraction. Lowering the weight forces the muscle to lengthen as it produces force, which is called an eccentric contraction. These lengthening muscle contractions have been shown to produce ultrastructural damage that may stimulate increased muscle protein turnover (*202*).

The effects of 52 weeks of high-intensity resistance training were examined in a group of 39 post-menopausal women (*203*). Twenty participants were randomly assigned to the strength training group (two days/week, 80% of 1RM for upper and lower body muscle groups). At the end of the year, significant differences were seen between the strength-trained and sedentary women in lumbar spine and femoral bone density. However, unlike other pharmacological and nutritional strategies for preventing bone loss and osteoporosis, resistance exercise affects more than just bone density. Women who engaged in strength training improved their muscle mass, strength, balance and overall levels of physical activity. Resistance training can thus be an important way to decrease the risk of an osteoporotic bone fracture in post-menopausal women.

Frontera et al. (*204*) examined the effects of high-intensity resistance training of the knee extensors and flexors (80% of 1RM, three days/week) in older men (aged 60–72). The average increase in knee flexor and extensor strength was 227% and 107%, respectively. Computed tomography scans and muscle biopsies were used to determine muscle size. Total muscle area by computed tomography analysis increased by 11.4% while the muscle biopsies showed a 33.5% increase in Type I fibre area and 27.5% increase in Type II fibre area. In addition, lower body VO2max increased significantly, while upper body VO2max did not, indicating that increased muscle mass can boost maximal aerobic power. It appears that the age-related loss in muscle mass may be an important determinant in the reduced maximal aerobic capacity seen in older men and women (*205*). Improving muscle strength can enhance the capacity of older men and women to perform many routine activities of daily living such as climbing stairs, carrying packages and even walking.

4.4 Interaction between exercise and supplementation

The same training approach was adopted in a group of frail institutionalized older men and women (mean age 90 ±3 years, range 87–96) (*206*). After eight weeks of training, the study's ten subjects had increased muscle strength by almost 180% and muscle size by 11%. More recently, a similar intervention (*207*) among frail nursing-home residents demonstrated not only increased muscle strength and size but also improved gait speed, stair-climbing power and balance. In addition, spontaneous activity levels increased significantly, while the activity of a non-exercising control group was unchanged. The study also examined the effects of combining exercise with a protein/calorie supplement—a 240 ml liquid supplying 360 $kcal_{th}$ in the form of carbohydrate (60%), fat (23%) and soy-based protein (17%)—which was designed to augment caloric intake by about 20% and provide one-third of the RDA for vitamins and minerals.

While no interaction was seen with muscle strength, functional capacity or muscle size, i.e. no differences were detected between the supplemented group and a non-supplemented controls, the men and women who consumed the supplement and exercised gained weight compared to the three other groups examined (exercise/control, non-exercise supplemented and non-exercise control). The non-exercising subjects who received the supplement reduced their habitual dietary energy intake so that total energy intake was unchanged. It is important to note that this was a very old, very frail population with diagnosed multiple chronic diseases. The increase in overall levels of physical activity has been a common observation in studies (*204, 203, 207*). Since muscle weakness is a primary deficit in many older individuals, increased strength may stimulate more aerobic activities such as walking and cycling.

The increased calorie requirements resulting from strength training may be a way for older persons to improve their overall nutritional intake when the calories are chosen as nutrient-dense foods. It is particularly important to increase intake of calcium, which was found to be one of the only limiting nutrients in the diet of free-living older men and women in the Boston Nutritional Status Survey for assessing free-living and institutionalized older men and women (*208*). Careful nutritional planning is needed to reach the recommended calcium levels of 1500 mg/day for post-menopausal women with osteoporosis or who are using hormone replacement therapy, and 1000 mg/day for post-menopausal women taking estrogen. Increased calorie intake from calcium-containing foods is one way to help achieve this goal.

In one of the few studies to examine the interaction of dietary calcium and exercise, 41 post-menopausal women consuming either high-calcium (1462 mg/day) or moderate-calcium (761 mg/day) diets were investigated. Half of these women participated in a yearlong walking program (45 minutes/day, 4 days/week, 75% of heart-rate reserve). Independent effects of the exercise and dietary calcium were seen. Compared with the moderate calcium group and irrespective of whether they exercised, the women consuming a high-calcium diet displayed reduced bone loss from the femoral neck. The walking prevented a loss of trabecular bone mineral density seen in the non-exercising women after one year. It thus appears that calcium intake and aerobic exercise are both independently beneficial to bone mineral density at different sites.

4.5 Recommendations

No group can benefit more than older persons from regularly performed exercise. Aerobic exercise has long been an important recommendation for preventing and treating many of the chronic and typically age-associated diseases. Moreover, research indicates that strength training is necessary both to stop or reverse sarcopenia and to increase bone density. Increasing muscle strength and mass in older persons is a realistic strategy for maintaining this group's functional status and independence. The following recommendations for aerobic and strength-training exercises are appropriate for individuals age 60 and older. Any exercise programme should, of course, always first be discussed with one's health care provider.

4.5.1 **Aerobic exercise**

Older persons should build up to at least 30 minutes of aerobic exercise—for example walking, swimming, water exercises and stationary cycling—on most, if not all, days.

4.5.2 **Strength training**

The following regimen allows the individual to maintain bone and muscle strength. In order to continue to strengthen muscle and bone, one should steadily increase the intensity (weight) of the workout. Recommendations are:

- Strength training 2 to 3 days a week, with a day of rest between workouts.
- In a fitness centre, 1 set of 8 to 12 repetitions on 12 or more machines.
- At home: 2 to 3 sets of 8 to 12 repetitions using 6 to 8 different exercises.
- When 12 repetitions can be made in good form with ease, weight lifted should be increased.

5. Assessing the nutritional status of older persons

5.1 Dietary intake

Dietary intake assessment, which is a key part of nutritional status analysis for both individuals and populations, is complicated for several reasons. Firstly, it is difficult to define appropriate samples representing various strata of the older population, e.g. free-living, homebound, institutionalized, healthy and sick. Secondly, the accuracy of nutrient-intake data is poor, especially in free-living older populations, because of limitations related to food-intake assessment methods and the completeness and accuracy of food composition tables. Thirdly, only a very limited number of controlled metabolic studies have been performed on older people to define requirements for several nutrients. Nevertheless, information on dietary intake is crucial and every effort should continue to be made to gather it. There are numerous methods including diet histories and recalls, diet records (kept by study participants or observed by research staff), and food-frequency question-naires. Choice of method depends on the goal of the study or survey, available personnel and funds, the literacy of the target population and cultural factors.

5.2 Body weight

Body weight is one of the least expensive physical measures to obtain. Weight can be compared to several standards to make a rough assessment of macronutrient status. Given the important relation between current weight and weight change in terms of predicting disability in older persons, today's weight can be compared to previous weight in an effort to estimate weight trajectory (209). Actual weight can then be compared to ideal weight based on actuarial data for the weight associated with lowest mortality (even if actuarial data, which are limited to middle-class, predominantly Caucasian, life-insurance applicants, may not be entirely representative of a given study population) (210). Next, it is possible to adjust weight-for-height using one of several possible body mass indices, e.g. the Quetelet index (kg/m^2). This is a simple and useful method with moderately good correlations ($r=0.6–0.8$) between BMI and fat mass and between BMI and lean mass (211). However, since the variability in fat (per cent of body fat) at a given BMI is extremely high and increases with age, predicting fat on the basis of BMI in an individual patient is very difficult to do (212, 213). It is because of this imprecision that assessment of the body compartments themselves is warranted.

5.3 **Body composition**

A range of techniques is available to assess trends in body composition over time. They include anthropometry and bioelectrical impedance (BIA), and more expensive and complex methods such as dual-energy X-ray absorptiometry, underwater weighing, isotope dilution or multicompartmental analysis with whole-body counting and neutron activation that can be used to determine fat and fat-free mass separately. As the technological sophistication of methods increases so, too, do their accuracy and cost, even as they become less widely available. For all practical purposes, assessment of the macronutrient status of large groups of older persons, whether free-living or in a clinical setting, still depends on BMI and less widely available anthropometry and BIA. It is important to begin by reviewing changes in body composition with ageing, as this can clarify the limitations of each of the measurement techniques. At the simplest level, body weight can be divided into fat mass and fat-free mass.

The precision and accuracy of body composition techniques correlates directly with their cost and inversely with their availability in a field or clinical setting. Anthropometry and BIA are the two methods most often available in such settings. From a strict technical perspective, both are flawed on theoretical grounds because they apply an oversimplified two-compartment model where body weight is partitioned into lean and fat. This approach is especially limited in older persons because the age-related decline in lean mass occurs preferentially in muscle, so that treating all the lean compartments—viscera, muscle and immune system—as a single whole lean is incorrect. Moreover, it means that the quality of the lean mass—the proportion that is muscle (*214*)—declines with age, and application of anthropometric or BIA equations that are derived from young people will give biased estimates of lean mass in older persons. In addition, since the estimate of lean mass is wrong, the error will propagate to the fat mass (since fat = weight – lean), and this compartment, too, will be measured inaccurately. Since the lean compartment is two to three times larger than the fat compartment in most people, the propagated error is proportionally much larger in the fat estimate than it is in the lean (see (*215*) for a review in this connection).

In addition to the theoretical problems related to these methods, there are also practical technical issues to consider. Firstly, anthropometry is very dependent on the skill of the operator, and there is often considerable inter-observer variability. Secondly, the commonly used equations that translate millimetres of skinfold and/or centimetres of circumference into kilograms of fat were generally developed for use with young, healthy adults and thus may not be accurate for older persons or ill populations. This problem is even more serious for BIA, which is critically dependent on the equation used. Moreover, it is very difficult to export equations from one population to another without introducing bias and imprecision (*216*). BIA's major advantage is that, unlike anthropometry, it is not operator-dependent and gives reproducible results over time. However, there are concerns, which are often ignored when data from populations are shown, about the method's accuracy when applied to individuals (*217*).

Despite these concerns, there is little doubt that some, even rudimentary, assessment of body compartments is better than no assessment at all. The important central issue is to use body composition data to help assess energy balance and macronutrient status in both patients and populations within the context of their physiologic and clinical situations. Unintentional weight loss, obesity, and current protein and fat content are all important clues to a person's health and physiologic age; they can be very helpful in both cross-sectional assessments—but especially in longitudinal assessments—of health and risk factors for disease, disability and mortality.

5.4 **Physical function**

There are abundant examples in the literature indicating that assessment of functional status, functional capacity, and exercise or physical capacity are useful predictors of survival, independence and disability (*218*). Functional status is generally a self-reported indication of a person's ability to perform tasks in his or her usual environment. As such, it incorporates elements of physical capacity to perform a task, environmental barriers (e.g. stairs, narrow doors or other impediments) to performing the task, and limitations on motivation (e.g. depression, dementia and loneliness). Functional status is generally measured by questionnaires, e.g. the WHO Questionnaire (*219*) or the Katz Activities of Daily Living Questionnaire (*220*). Because of the self-reported nature of functional status, it is susceptible to all the biases and imprecision of any questionnaire-based instrument. It nevertheless remains valid to the degree that self-reporting is a reflection of a person's own perception of his or her current state.

In contrast, functional capacity is a laboratory or field-based measurement of a subject's ability to perform such tasks as rising from a chair, balancing and walking at a fast pace. Various measures of varying degrees of sophistication, duration and complexity have been developed to assess functional capacity. For example, some tests measure simple tasks as described above, while others involve more complex or instrumental activities such as putting on a sweater, shopping or using a telephone. Obviously, these tests have to be culturally appropriate, which complicates comparison of results between countries. However, many basic tasks such as rising from a seated position, tandem and semi-tandem gait, and gait speed are universal and can be applied to very disparate cultures.

Measurements of exercise capacity such as maximal strength (1RM or other methods) or oxygen carrying capacity (VO2max), which generally require specialized equipment and are not easily performed in field settings, are not considered here.

5.5 **Immune function**

Records of episodes among older persons of common infectious illness, e.g. upper respiratory tract infection, pneumonia, urinary tract infection and diarrhoea, are one approach to assessing body defences. If affordable, DTH is helpful in evaluating cellular immunity in addition to having prognostic significance in terms of mortality. The total lymphocyte count from a blood film, which can also be used as an index of immune function, is readily accessible at the second and third levels of a three-level classification of health services. When performed in the community, testing antibody levels following vaccination can be a useful immune indicator. Other tests of immune function are unlikely to be available or affordable to either the majority of older persons or their caregivers.

5.6 **Other laboratory indices**

Biomarkers of food intake are attractive for assessing the nutritional status of individuals and communities. However, it is unusual that intake of a given food component will explain even 50% of the variance in blood, urine or tissue levels of that nutrient/food component on a given day. In any case, biomarkers are more likely to indicate various genetic food-intake and lifestyle factors, which may be useful in their own right. Availability and cost are overriding considerations. Simple haematological indices of haemoglobin and blood film remain invaluable and cost-effective. Low-technology dry-chemistry techniques now available to assess metabolic disorders (as with glycaemic and lipid disorders) are becoming realistic options given the shift towards chronic NCDs in disease patterns among older persons.

5.7 **Community variables**

In addition to clinical tests, functional status and the anthropometric assessments that form the basis of strategies for improving the health of older adults, assessment of a variety of other parameters is useful for defining interventions. For example, understanding the cultural, social and economic factors that influence the nutritional and health status of older persons in a given community is vital to designing appropriate educational messages and programmes. At the same time, a review of community assets can be helpful in creating programmes and campaigns and developing projection methods. Literacy levels of older persons, their living situations, availability of adequate and safe food resources, cooking facilities and transportation options all need to be considered when designing strategies for behavioural change. Finally, assessing the presence and capacity of community-based agencies and organizations regarding nutrition and related activities allows health promotion experts to maximize the impact of programmes while avoiding any duplication of efforts.

5.8 Summary of assessment techniques

The following should be considered a minimum set of assessments for establishing the nutritional and functional status of older populations:

- Dietary information
- Weight
- Height
- Waist circumference
- Mid-arm circumference
- Subcutaneous skinfold
- Functional status (questionnaire)
- Infection episodes (questionnaire)

A second group of more sophisticated tests may be added if resources permit:

- Bioelectrical impedance
- Short physical performance battery (altered as culturally appropriate)
- Delayed-type hypersensitivity testing
- Chemical markers
- Antibody levels following vaccination when performed in the community

6. Nutritional guidelines for healthy ageing

6.1 Food-based dietary guidelines

It is clear that a wide variety of food cultures and cuisines are consistent with, and can help to promote, healthy ageing. The traditional nutrient-based approach was limited in that it did not take into account the environmental, social, economic and lifestyle context of eating. It also did not adequately deal with the chemical complexity of foods and the interaction and synergies between foods and food components. Considering diet and health relationships in a culturally sensitive way and providing consumers with easier ways to make healthy food choices is the foundation of the food-based dietary guideline approach (Annex 3) that FAO and WHO have been promoting since 1996 (221).

6.2 Nutrient intake recommendations for older persons

There are many questions about how best to define nutrient requirements for older persons. Previously, biochemical standards and balance studies often served as the gold standard for assessing nutrient requirements. However, homeostatic adaptation can severely limit the usefulness of this approach, particularly for assessing certain minerals and vitamin A. Rather than merely knowing the amount of nutrient it takes to prevent a *deficiency state*, gerontologists and nutritionists are also interested in the amount of nutrient that it takes to prevent a *chronic disease* from occurring. In some cases, e.g. osteoporosis, there are sufficient data on how much of a nutrient it takes to affect either a marker of chronic disease or a chronic disease itself. Reliable data, derived directly from experiments conducted with older persons, are available on nutritional requirements for older persons for the following nutrients.

6.2.1 *Energy*

Since low levels of physical activity and unchanged levels of energy absorption typically accompany older age, lower energy intakes are required to prevent obesity. Nevertheless, Roberts et al. have shown an underestimation of the amount of energy expenditure required for routine physical activities associated with daily living (222). These investigators calculate that the total energy expenditure to resting energy expenditure ratio is ~1.75 (versus the 1.5 figure on which the 1989 RDAs in the USA are based) (63). Impaired capacity, possibly associated with increased body fat, for energy expenditure to adapt to short-term changes (whether positive or negative) in energy intake has also been demonstrated in older individuals

(*223*). If energy requirements have been underestimated in previous studies of older persons, protein requirements may have been overestimated in nitrogen balance experiments. In order to make more accurate estimates of the raw energy requirements of ageing, consensus needs to be reached on the desirable range of physical activity for older people. Pending final resolution of these issues, the energy requirements of old age appear to be 1.4 to 1.8 multiples of the BMR to maintain body weight at different levels of physical activity. Levels of physical activity that result in energy requirements in the higher end of the range are desirable for reducing morbidity and mortality.

6.2.2 *Calcium*

An age-related decrease in calcium absorption—probably due to changes in vitamin D metabolism—has been demonstrated in humans. Since atrophic gastritis results in reduced gastric acid, the effect of gastric acidity on calcium bioavailability has also been investigated. No acid-related effect has been found on the bioavailability of calcium from a meal (*224*).

Inadequate calcium ingestion has been documented in many populations of older persons around the world. Several large-scale intervention studies have been completed in an attempt to arrive at a calcium requirement for older persons based on the effect of calcium intakes on bone mineral loss (*225–227*). These studies were conducted using calcium supplements with a diverse range of dietary calcium intakes. In some studies vitamin D supplementation was also provided. Thus, for example, it is not possible to know from available data the exact amount of calcium needed to prevent bone mineral loss in older women. In the presence of adequate vitamin D nutrition, it appears that calcium intakes in the range of 800–1200 mg/day will result in both a beneficial effect on bone mineral density of the femur, neck and lumbar spine and a reduction in fracture rates. Potential benefits of high calcium intakes and various other health-related measures, e.g. reduced blood pressure and decreased risk of a colon cancer, may also be important, although data are insufficient to know for certain.

6.2.3 *Copper*

Ageing has not been associated with significant changes in copper metabolism, and copper balance has been maintained in older people at dietary intakes of about 1.3 mg/day (*228*). The WHO recommendation for dietary copper intake, including for persons over 60 years of age, is 1.3 mg/day (*229*). An intake of 1.3–1.5 mg/day should thus be adequate for older persons (*230*).

6.2.4 *Chromium*

Chromium acts as a co-factor for insulin and is required for normal lipid and glucose metabolism. Chromium supplementation of 200–250 μg/day has resulted in some improvement in glucose tolerance, insulin response and blood lipids in older populations (*231, 232*). However, chromium balance in older adults can be achieved with dietary chromium intakes of < 50 µg/day (*233*).

6.2.5 *Fat*

Except where overweight or obesity are problems, there is no further health benefit from restricting fat calories in older persons beyond 30% for sedentary, and 35% for active, older persons (*234*). However, consumption of saturated fats should be minimized and not exceed 8% of total energy. It is desirable to have a variety of fats in the diet, particularly an adequate intake of the ω-3 fatty acids found in fish, soy, linseed, canola seed and oil, seaweed and green leaves.

6.2.6 *Folate*

In 1979 Jagerstad & Westesson reported from Sweden that among 35 older persons with a mean folate intake of about 100–200 µg/day, all 35 had normal whole-blood folate levels over a period of 16 years (*235*). On the basis of a serum folate cut-off value of 3.0 µg/ml (*236*), the Boston Nutritional Status Survey determined that less than 2.5% of either free-living or institutionalized older persons studied were deficient. In past efforts to set recommended dietary intake levels for folate, both macrocytic anaemia and serum folate values have been used as indicators of folate deficiency. These observations may have contributed to unjustified confidence about the adequacy of folate status among older persons.

More recently, however, a new marker of folate status—homocysteine levels—has come into widespread use. Selhub et al. found that homocysteine values in blood were elevated when serum folate levels were lower than 5.0 µg/ml (*237*). If a 5.0 µg/ml cut-off had been used in the Boston Survey, 15% of older persons would have been defined as deficient (*236*). There is great interest in the role of homocysteine as an atherogenic agent and the possibility that tissue folate deficiency could play an indirect role in atheromatous disease. Data from the Framingham Heart Study among older people demonstrated that serum homocysteine levels are correlated with dietary folate levels, and that serum homocysteine levels are high at dietary intakes of < 400 µg/day (*237*). Red blood cell folate levels are also maintained at this level of folate intake. Large-scale intervention studies will be needed to show that administration of folate at this level or above will in fact diminish the risk of vascular disease.

6.2.7 *Iron*

Haem iron absorption is not affected by ageing. In addition, non-haem iron has not been found to be different in healthy older persons compared to healthy young men. Some surveys have reported that serum ferritin concentrations in older men increase with age, although other studies have not found this relationship. However, serum ferritin levels in older persons are difficult to interpret since inflammation can elevate serum ferritin (*238*). No relationship between age and serum ferritin has been observed in studies of older persons selected to be free of inflammation and/or diseases known to alter serum ferritin concentrations (*239*).

Since iron is a pro-oxidant nutrient, additional research is required on whether there is progressive body iron accumulation with ageing, and on possible linkages between iron status and chronic disease. Pending completion of further studies of older populations, and on the assumption that there are no excessive iron losses, e.g. from hookworm or schistosomiasis, it appears that 10 mg/day is an adequate intake for older men and women.

6.2.8 *Magnesium*
Dietary intakes of magnesium have been estimated in western countries to be between 225–280 mg for persons over the age of 65 (*230*). In the absence of compelling evidence that magnesium deficiency is prevalent in western society, this appears to be an adequate intake level.

6.2.9 *Protein*
The results of various studies on protein balance are difficult to compare since different nitrogen balance formulas were used and different assumptions were applied to the calculations. Campbell et al. recently assessed nitrogen balance data from four studies of older persons and determined, by combined weighted averaging, that the overall protein requirement for older persons is 0.91 ± 0.04 g/kg per day (*240*). This is higher than the 0.75 g protein/kg per day recommended by the 1985 FAO/WHO/UNU consultation (*64*).

Castenada et al. recently completed a study assessing long-term adaptation to marginal protein intakes in 12 older women (66–79 years) (*241*). The subjects' diets contained either 0.45 or 0.92 g protein/kg per day, and their nitrogen balance was measured. All women on the 0.45 g protein/kg per day diet were in negative balance, but the mean negative nitrogen balance moved significantly towards nitrogen equilibrium at week nine. However, this shift was accompanied by an 8% decline in body cell mass. In contrast, the women eating 0.92 g/kg per day showed an increase in their muscle mass and insulin-like growth factor-1 levels, suggesting that this level of protein was more than adequate (*241*). From this study, a mean protein requirement of 0.78 g/protein/kg per day for nitrogen equilibrium was estimated via a regression analysis from both the low- and high-protein diets (*240*). In general, protein intakes of 0.9–1.1 g/kg per day may be considered beneficial for healthy older persons.

6.2.10 *Riboflavin*
Boisvert et al. recently studied riboflavin-depleted older persons and gradually repleted them with increasing amounts of dietary riboflavin (*242*). The slope of

urinary riboflavin excretion rose sharply when dietary intake reached 1.1 mg per day, which is the identical level at which the slope of the riboflavin-excretion curve changed in a classic study of younger adults (*243*). Thus, despite lower energy expenditure in older people, riboflavin requirements appear to be the same as for younger people. The RDA for the 19–70 age range is 1.3 mg/day for men and 1.1. mg/day for women. Contrary to earlier assumptions, there is no evidence that older people have diminished riboflavin requirements.

6.2.11 **Selenium**

Several studies have shown low serum or plasma selenium concentrations in adults over 60 years of age compared to younger adults. In one study in the United Kingdom, selenium intakes in housebound older persons (70–85 years) were approximately 38 µg/day (*244*). Despite this low mean intake, older persons remained in positive selenium balance. Based on available data, it appears that 50–70 µg/day of selenium should be more than adequate for older persons (*230*).

6.2.12 **Vitamin B12**

While it is known that many older persons absorb poorly protein-bound vitamin B12, absorption of crystalline vitamin B12 proceeds normally. For example, Carmel reported on 47 patients with low serum vitamin B12 concentrations who had normal Schilling tests of vitamin B12 absorption when the crystalline vitamin was used as the test dose (*245*). However, when protein-bound vitamin B12 absorption tests were performed, 42% had abnormally low results. Many of the patients with malabsorption of protein-bound vitamin B12 had atrophic gastritis, a prevalent condition in older people affecting 10–30% of Americans over the age of 60 (*246, 247*). The much greater prevalence of atrophic gastritis, which is particularly high in China and certain South American countries, is believed to be related to chronic stomach infection with *Helicobactor pylori* (*248*). The mechanism of protein-bound vitamin B12 malabsorption in atrophic gastritis involves both maldigestion of the food protein-vitamin B12 complex in the stomach and the uptake of any free vitamin B12 by the large number of bacteria that proliferate in the low-acid conditions found in the stomach (*249*).

There is no evidence that, once absorbed, vitamin B12 is metabolized differently in older persons than in younger people. Moreover, as stated above, crystalline vitamin B12 can be absorbed normally even in the presence of atrophic gastritis. Thus, in order to cover the needs of older persons with atrophic gastritis, the recommendation should be to meet vitamin B12 requirements (2.5 µg/day) either by taking a vitamin B12 supplement or by eating vitamin B12-fortified foods (*250*). There is no evidence that vitamin B12 requirements change with age. Policy-makers should consider the need for food fortification in general and make specific dietary recommendations to ensure that older persons can meet their vitamin B12 requirements.

6.2.13 *Vitamin A*

The RDA for vitamin A was set high in the USA in 1989 due to the possible role of provitamin carotenoids in disease prevention, e.g. cancer, cardiovascular disease. β-carotene and certain other carotenoids are vitamin A precursors. However, three intervention studies have shown that high levels of β-carotene, taken alone, not only do not reduce the risk of cancer or cardiovascular disease; they also, in fact, increase the incidence of lung carcinoma in heavy smokers (*15, 251, 252*). Moreover, concern has been expressed about a low margin of safety for preformed dietary vitamin A in older persons since higher serum retinyl ester values occur in older people than in younger people who have been exposed to identical vitamin A-containing supplements (*253*). Higher retinyl ester levels are thought to be the result of either increased vitamin A absorption by the older gastrointestinal tract and/or decreased plasma clearance of retinyl esters and chylomicron remnants by the liver. The Seneca study reported a high prevalence of vitamin A intakes below the lowest European recommended dietary intake (700 µg retinol equivalents (RE) for males and 600 µg RE for females) (*254*). For example in Chateau Renault-Amboise (France), despite 80% of older males having dietary intakes of < 700 µg/day, none of the subjects had deficient serum vitamin A values. In other studies, no effect of age alone on hepatic concentrations was found in the 66 to 96 age range (*255*). Based on these considerations, it appears that 600–700 µg RE/day represents an adequate intake for older men and women.

6.2.14 *Vitamin C*

Many studies have reported age-related declines in serum ascorbic acid concentrations; however, the pharmokinetics of a 500 mg oral dose of vitamin C are no different between older and younger men (*256*). Moreover, in a depletion study, the half-life of the depletion stage was found to be the same in older as in younger people (*257*). Vanderjagt et al. showed that a dietary intake of 150mg/day would be needed to maintain a plasma concentration of 1.0 mg/dl (the level corresponding to the maximal body pool) in older men, and that 80 mg/day would be required for older women (*258*). However, it is uncertain what health benefits would accrue from maintaining a plasma concentration at which body pools are saturated.

High vitamin C blood levels and/or intakes have been associated with a lower prevalence of senile cataract, higher high-density lipoprotein cholesterol concentrations and lower incidences of coronary artery disease (*259–261*). These areas of investigation should of course be pursued. For now, however, it appears that older persons do not have different vitamin C requirements to younger people and that an intake level of 60–100 mg/day is adequate (*63*).

6.2.15 *Vitamin D*

There are many reasons for vitamin D malnutrition in older persons including low exposure to sunlight, poor skin response to sunlight, and decreased absorption or decreased hydroxylation of vitamin D. Fish and meat are important sources of this vitamin in many countries, and in the USA vitamin D-fortified milk is a principal source. There is great interest in the amount of dietary vitamin D needed to prevent bone demineralization. Dawson-Hughes et al. investigated vitamin D in bone loss in 249 healthy postmenopausal women in Boston (42°N latitude) (*262, 263*). The women were randomly assigned to receive 10 µg of vitamin D per day or a placebo in addition to their usual dietary intake of 2.5 µg. All received a calcium supplement of about 400 mg/day in addition to a mean dietary calcium intake of 400 mg/day. Spine and whole-body mineral density was assessed using dual energy X-ray absorptiometry. It was found that wintertime bone loss was greatly reduced in volunteers taking the 10 µg vitamin D supplement. Previously, it had been shown that 1.2 g of elemental calcium and 20 µg of vitamin D/day significantly reduced the risk of hip fractures in older women (*263*). Similar findings have been reported from the USA. Based on available studies, it appears that older persons need 10–20 µg vitamin D per day to ensure optimal bone health (*250*).

6.2.16 *Vitamin E*

Most of the interest in vitamin E requirements has centred on the possible beneficial effects of pharmacological doses (60–400 IU/day) of the vitamin, which could not be achieved through an otherwise healthy diet and which have been shown to improve several indicators of immune status (*264*). Vitamin E is of interest as a protective antioxidant and membrane stabilizer. In addition, a relation has been demonstrated between high circulating vitamin E concentrations or vitamin E supplementation use and lower prevalence of cataract and cancer (*265, 266*). High doses of vitamin E may also play a role in slowing the progression of Alzheimer disease (*267*), while a 100–400 IU/day dose has been shown to prevent cardio-vascular disease. However, only one intervention study has shown a secondary prevention effect (*268*), and only one other study has shown a slight primary prevention effect (*269*). Further research is needed to determine the adequacy of current vitamin E recommendations for older persons.

6.2.17 *Vitamin K*

Several studies have shown that older persons have significantly higher plasma phylloquinione concentrations than younger adults (*270, 271*). In some cases, higher levels of triglyceride-rich lipoproteins, with advancing age, can account for these higher concentrations. Ferland et al. have shown a resistance among older adults in functional measures of vitamin K deficiency when placed on low vitamin K diets (*262*). This is probably due to greater vitamin K intake among older versus younger adults. For now, vitamin K intake in the 60–90 mg range appears to be adequate for older people. The role of vitamin K in bone mineralization remains an important area of investigation.

6.2.18 *Zinc*

Various studies have shown dietary intakes of zinc among healthy older people ranging from 5.8 to 12.8 mg/day. However, as with iron, more reliable indicators of zinc status are needed in older persons before definitive judgements can be made about the state of this group's zinc nutriture. Zinc status is especially important for older persons, who need to maintain their full immunocompetence. Based on available data, the following are recommended nutrient intakes for dietary zinc for people over 65 years of age:

High Zn availability (> 50%):	Men	4.2 mg/day
	Women	3.0 mg/day
Moderate Zn availability (30%):	Men	7.0 mg/day
	Women	4.9 mg/day
Low Zn availability (15%):	Men	14.0 mg/day
	Women	9.8 mg/day

6.2.19 *Phytochemicals*

In addition to the recognized essential nutrients, there are many other food components—collectively known as phytochemicals—about which little is known but whose biological effects can lower the risk of major health problems such as cancer and heart disease. Their effects may be hormonal, anti-inflammatory, anti-microbial, anti-oxidant, anti-mutagenic or anti-angiogenic. For this reason alone it is important to obtain essential nutrients through a food-based approach and not be dependent on vitamin and mineral supplements. Research to identify the presence and role of these phytochemicals in the diets of older people should be given high priority. The potential health-promoting aspects of phytochemicals should also be considered in terms of agricultural and trade policies and strategies. Modern agricultural and aquacultural practices frequently alter—whether positively or negatively—the composition of traditional foods. These, too, may have important implications for nutritional recommendations for older persons.

6.2.20 *Other dietary considerations*

There is a need for more complete documentation of diet-health relationships throughout the life course that looks beyond deficiency disorders. To promote health messages in geographically and culturally diverse populations, researchers should examine food components and dietary constituents that are associated with positive long-term biological effects.

References

1. *World Population Prospects: the 2000 revision (medium variant)*. NewYork, United Nations, Population Division, 2001.

2. *World Population Prospects: the 1998 revision (medium variant)*. NewYork, United Nations, Population Division, 1999.

3. Steen B, Landin I, Mellström D. Nutrition and health in the eighth decade of life. In: Wahlqvist M et al., eds. *Nutrition in a sustainable environment*. London, Smith-Gordon, 1994:331–333.

4. Khaw KT. Healthy ageing. *British Medical Journal*, 1997, **315**:1090–1096.

5. Kalache A, Ebrahim S, eds. *Epidemiology in Old Age*. London, BMJ Publishing Group, 1996.

6. Andrews GR et al., eds. *Ageing in the Western Pacific—A four-country study*. Manila, Regional Office of the World Health Organization, 1986 (Western Pacific Reports and Studies No.1).

7. De Groot LCPGM, van Staveren WA, Hautvast JGAJ. Euronut-SENECA. Nutrition and the elderly in Europe. *European Journal of Clinical Nutrition*, 1991, **45**:S3.

8. *International classification of functioning and disability*. Geneva, World Health Organization, 2001 (Internet: http://who.int/classification/icf).

9. Wahlqvist ML, Savige GS, Lukito W. Nutritional disorders in the elderly. *Medical Journal of Australia*, 1995, **163**:376–381.

10. Lucas A. Programming by early nutrition: an experimental approach. *Journal of Nutrition*, 1998, **128**:401S–406S.

11. Barker DJ. Maternal nutrition and cardiovascular disease. *Nutrition and Health*, 1993, **2**:99–106.

12. Barker DJ et al. The relation of small head circumference and thinness at birth to death from cardiovascular disease in adult life. *British Medical Journal*, 1993, **306**(6875): 422–426.

13. Barker DJ. The intrauterine origins of cardiovascular disease. *Acta Paediatrica Supplement*, 1993, **82**, S391:93–99.

14. Heaney RP. The role of nutrition in prevention and management of osteoporosis. *Clinical Obstetrics and Gynecology*, 1987, **50**:833–846.

15. The Alpha-Tocopherol, Beta Carotene Cancer Prevention Study Group. The effect of vitamin E and beta carotene on the incidence of lung cancer and other cancers in male smokers. *New England Journal of Medicine*, 1994, **330**:1029–1035.

16. MacLennan R et al. Randomized trial of intake of fat, fibre, and beta carotene to prevent colorectal adenomas. *Journal of the National Cancer Institute*, 1995, **87**:1760–1766.

17. Pan XR et al. Effects of diet and exercise in preventing NIDDM in people with impaired glucose tolerance. The Da Qing IGT and Diabetes Study. *Diabetes Care*, 1997, **20**:537–544.

18. Salmeron J et al. Dietary fibre, glycaemic load, and risk of non-insulin-dependent diabetes mellitus in women. *Journal of the American Medical Association*, 1997, **277**:472–477.

19. Feskens EJ et al. Dietary factors determining diabetes and impaired glucose tolerance. A 20-year follow-up of the Finnish and Dutch cohorts of the Seven Countries Study. *Diabetes Care*, 1995, **18**:1104–1112.

20. Wahlqvist ML. Nutrition and diabetes. *Australian Family Physician*, 1997, **26**:384–389.

21. Pan DA et al. Skeletal muscle membrane lipid composition is related to adiposity and insulin action. *Journal of Clinical Investigation*, 1995, **96**:2802–2808.

22. Jain SK et al. Effect of modest vitamin E supplementation on blood glycated hemoglobin and triglyceride levels and red cell indices in Type I diabetic patients. *Journal of the American College of Nutrition*, 1996, **15**:458–461.

23. Jovanovic-Peterson L, Peterson CM. Vitamin and mineral deficiencies which may predispose to glucose intolerance of pregnancy. *Journal of the American College of Nutrition*, 1996, **15**:14–20.

24. Goulding A et al. Sodium and osteoporosis. In: Wahlqvist ML, Truswell AS, eds. *Recent advances in clinical nutrition*. London, John Libby, 1986:99–108.

25. Dalais F et al. Effects of dietary phytoestrogens in postmenopausal women. *Climacteric*, 1998, **1**:124–129.

26. Kuiper GG et al. Comparison of the ligand binding specificity and transcript tissue distribution of estrogen receptors alpha and beta. *Endocrinology*, 1997, **138**:863–870.

27. Littlejohn GO, Wahlqvist ML. The use of unproven remedies for arthritis. *General Practitioner*, 1993, **1**:68 and 1993, **1**:8–9.

28. Kestin M et al. The use of unproven remedies for rheumatoid arthritis in Australia. *Medical Journal of Australia*, 1985, **143**:516–518.

29. Landrum JT, Bone RA, Kilburn MD. The macular pigment: a possible role in protection from age-related macular degeneration. *Advanced Pharmacology*, 1997, **38**:537–556.

30. Seddon JM et al. Dietary carotenoids, vitamins A, C, and E, and advanced age-related macular degeneration. Eye Disease Case-Control Study Group. *Journal of the American Medical Association*, 1994, **272**:1413–1420.

31. Prinsley DM, Sandstead HH. *Nutrition and Ageing*. New York, Alan R. Liss Inc., 1990.

32. Evans JG, Williams TF. *Oxford textbook of geriatric medicine*. Oxford, New York: Oxford University Press, 1992.

33. Kuczmarski RJ et al. Increasing prevalence of overweight among U.S. adults. The National Health and Nutrition Examination Surveys, 1960 to 1991. *Journal of the American Medical Association*, 1994, **272**:205–211.

34. Frontera WR, Hughes VA, Evans WJ. A cross-sectional study of upper and lower extremity muscle strength in 45–78 year old men and women. *Journal of Applied Physiology*, 1991, **71**:644–650.

35. Moore FD. Energy and the maintenance of body cell mass. *Journal of Parenteral Nutrition*, 1980, **4**:228–260.

36. Krieger M. Ueber die Atrophie der menschlichen Organe bei Inanition. [On human atrophy as a result of under-nutrition.] *Z. Angew. Anat. Konstitutionsl.*, 1921, **7**:87–134.

37. Winick M. *Hunger disease-studies by Jewish physicians in the Warsaw ghetto*. New York, John Wiley & Sons, 1979.

38. Kotler DP, Tierney AR, Pierson RN. Magnitude of body cell mass depletion and the timing of death from wasting in AIDS. *American Journal of Clinical Nutrition*, 1989, **50**:444–447.

39. Flynn MA et al. Total body potassium in ageing humans: A longitudinal study. *American Journal of Clinical Nutrition*, 1989, **50**:713–717.

40. Cohn SH et al. Compartmental body composition based on total-body nitrogen, potassium, and calcium. *American Journal of Physiology*, 1980, **239**:E524–E530.

41. Freeman LM, Roubenoff R. The nutrition implications of cardiac cachexia. *Nutrition Reviews*, 1994, **52**:340–347.

42. Dinarello CA, Roubenoff R. Mechanisms of loss of lean body mass in patients with chronic dialysis. *Blood Purification*, 1996, **14**:388–394.

43. Caregaro L et al. Malnutrition in alcoholic and virus-related cirrhosis. *American Journal of Clinical Nutrition*,1996, **63**:602–609.

44. Nielsen K et al. Nutritional assessment and adequacy of dietary intake in hospitalized patients with alcoholic liver cirrhosis. *British Journal of Nutrition*, 1993, **69**:665–679.

45. King AJ et al. Cytokine production and nutritional status hemodialysis patients. *International Journal of Artificial Organs*, 1998, **21**:4–11.

46. Roubenoff R et al. Rheumatoid cachexia: cytokine-driven hypermetabolism and loss of lean body mass in chronic inflammation. *Journal of Clinicial Investigation*, 1994, **93**:2397–2386.

47. Roubenoff R et al. Rheumatoid cachexia: Depletion of lean body mass in rheumatoid arthritis. Possible association with rumor necrosis factor. *Journal of Rheumatology*, 1992, **19**:1505–1510.

48. Roubenoff R et al. Standardization of nomenclature of body composition in weight loss. *American Journal of Clinical Nutrition*, 1997, **66**:192–196.

49. Roubenoff R, Harris TB. Failure to thrive, sarcopenia and functional decline in the elderly. *Clinical Geriatric Medicine*, 1997, **13**:613–622.

50. Pelleymounter MA et al. Effects of the obese gene product on body weight regulation in ob/ob mice. *Science*, 1995, **269**:540–543.

51. Ronnemaa T et al. Relation between plasma leptin levels and measures of body fat in identical twins discordant for obesity. *Annals of Internal Medicine*, 1997, **126**:26–31.

52. Roubenoff R et al. The relationship between growth hormone kinetics and sarcopenia in postmenopausal women: the role of fat mass and leptin. *Journal of Clinicial Endocrinology and Metabolism*, 1998, **83**:1502–1506.

53. National Institutes of Health Consensus Development Panel on the Health Implications of Obesity. Health Implications of Obesity. *Annals of Internal Medicine*, 1985, **103**:1073–1077.

54. Dawson-Hughes B et al. Effect of calcium and vitamin D supplementation on bone density in men and women 65 years of age or older. *New England Journal of Medicine*, 1997, **337**:670–676.

55. Chapuy MC et al. Vitamin D3 and calcium to prevent hip fractures in elderly women. *New England Journal of Medicine*, 1992, **327**:1637–1642.

56. US Department of Health and Human Services, National Center for Health Statistics. *Dietary intake source data: United States, 1976–80*. Washington, DC, US Government Printing Office, DHHS publication (PHS) 1983:83–1681.

57. DiPietro L et al. Depressive symptoms and weight change in a national cohort of adults. *International Journal of Obesity*, 1992, **16**:745–753.

58. Morley JE, Silver A J. Anorexia in the elderly. *Neurobiological Ageing*, 1988, **9**:9–16.

59. Arora S et al. Effect of age on tests of intestinal and hepatic function in healthy humans. *Gastroenterology*, 1998, **9**:1560–1565.

60. Durnin JVGA. Low energy expenditures in free-living populations. *European Journal of Clinical Nutrition*, 1990, **4**:95–102.

61. Roberts SB et al. Influence of age on energy requirements. *American Journal of Clinical Nutrition*, 1995, **62**:1053S–1058S.

62. Roberts SB et al. Impaired control of food intake in older men. *Journal of the American Medical Association*, 1994, **272**:1601–1606.

63. National Research Council. *Recommended dietary allowances, 10th edition*. Washington DC, National Academy Press, 1989.

64. *Energy and protein requirements. Report of a joint FAO/WHO/UNU Expert Consultation*. Geneva, World Health Organization, 1986 (WHO Technical Report Series, No. 724).

65. Shaffer SE, Tepper BJ. Effects of learned flavor cues on single meal and daily food intake in humans. *Physiological Behaviour*, 1994, **55**:979–986.

66. Arvidson K. Location and variation in the number of taste buds in human fungiform papillae. *Scandinavian Journal of Dental Research*, 1979, **87**:435–442.

67. Bastoshuk LM, Rifkin B, Marks LE. Taste and ageing. *Journal of Gerontology*, 1986, **41**:51–57.

68. Kamath, SK. Taste acuity and ageing. *American Journal of Clinical Nutrition*, 1982, **36**:766–775.

69. Alaria E. Investigations on the human taste organs. I. The structure of the taste papillae at various ages. *Archivio Italiano di Anatomia e di Embriologia* [*Italian Archives of Anatomy and Embryology*], 1939, **49**:506–514.

70. Schiffman SS, Warwick ZS. Effect of flavor enhancement of foods for the elderly on nutritional status: food intake, biochemical indices, and anthropometric measures. *Physiological Behaviour*, 1993, **53**:395–402.

71. Doty RL et al. Smell identification ability: changes with age. *Science*, 1984, **226**:1441–1443.

72. Morley JE. Anorexia of ageing: physiologic and pathologic. *American Journal of Clinical Nutrition*, 1997, **66**:760–773.

73. Schiffman SS, Gatlin CA. Clinical physiology of taste and smell. *Annual Review of Nutrition*, 1993, **13**:405–436.

74. Drewnowski A et al. Salt taste perceptions and preferences are unrelated to consumption in healthy older adults. *Journal of the American Dietetic Association*, 1996, **96**:471–474.

75. Weinberg AD, Minaker KL. Dehydration. Evaluation and management in older adults. Council on Scientific Affairs, American Medical Association. *Journal of the American Medical Association*, 1995, **274**:1552–1556.

76. Reyes-Ortiz CA. Dehydration, delirium, and disability in elderly persons. *Journal of the American Medical Association*, 1997, **278**:287–288.

77. Ferruci L et al. Hospital diagnoses, Medicare charges, and nursing home admissions in the year when older persons become severely disabled. *Journal of the American Medical Association*, 1997, **278**:728–734.

78. Phillips PA et al. Reduced thirst after water deprivation in healthy elderly men. *New England Journal of Medicine*, 1984, **311**:753–759.

79. Mack GW et al. Body fluid balance in dehydrated healthy older men: thirst and renal osmoregulation. *Journal of Applied Physiology*, 1994, **76**:1615-1623.

80. Silver AJ, Morley JE. Role of the opioid system in the hypodypsia associated with ageing. *Journal of the American Geriatric Society*, 1992, **40**:556–560.

81. Crane MG, Harris JJ. Effect of ageing on renin activity and aldosterone excretion. *Journal of the Laboratory of Clinical Medicine*, 1976, **87**: 947–959.

82. Kirkland J et al. Plasma arginine vasopressin in dehydrated elderly patients. *Clinical Endocrinology*, 1984, **20**:451–456.

83. Stachenfeld NS et al. Thirst and fluid regulatory responses to hypertonicity in older adults. *American Journal of Physiology*, 1996, **271**:R757–R765.

84. Stachenfeld NS et al. Mechanism of attenuated thirst in ageing: role of central volume receptors. *American Journal of Physiology*, 1997, **272**:R148–R157.

85. Warren JL, Harris T, Phillips C. Dehydration in older adults. *Journal of the American Medical Association*, 1996, **275**:912.

86. Johnson RH et al. Effect of posture on blood pressure in elderly patients. *Lancet*, 1965, **1**:731–733.

87. Berger EY. Nutrition by hypodermoclysis. *Journal of the American Geriatric Society*, 1984, **32**:199–203.

88. Chidester JC, Spangler AA. Fluid intake in the institutionalized elderly. *Journal of the American Dietetic Association*, 1997, **97**:23–28.

89. Miller RA. Accumulation of hyporesponsive, calcium extruding memory T cells as a key feature of age-dependent immune dysfunction. *Clinical Immunology and Immunopathology*, 1991, **58**:305–317.

90. Wayne SJ et al. Cell-mediated immunity as a predictor of morbidity and mortality in the aged. *Journal of Gerontological Science*, 1990, **45**:M45–M48.

91. Christou NV et al. Estimating mortality risk in preoperative patients using immunologic, nutritional, and acute-phase response variables. *Annals of Surgery*, 1989, **210**:69–77.

92. Cohn JR, Hohl CA, Buckley CE. The relationship between cutaneous cellular immune responsiveness and mortality in a nursing home population. *Journal of the American Geriatric Society*, 1983, **31**:808–809.

93. Abbas AK, Lichtman AH, Pober JS. *Cellular and molecular immunology*. Philadelphia, W.B. Saunders Company, 1991.

94. Makinodan T, Hirokawa K. Normal ageing of the immune system. In: Johnson HA, ed. *Relations between normal ageing and disease*. New York, Raven Press, 1985:117–132.

95. Green-Johnson J, Wade AW, Szewczuk MR. The immunobiology of ageing. In: Cooper EL, Nisbet-Brown E, eds. *Developmental immunology*. New York, Oxford University Press, 1993:426–451.

96. Miller RA. Cellular and biochemical changes in the ageing mouse immune system. *Nutrition Reviews*, 1995, **53**:S14–S17.

97. Schwab R, Weksler ME. Cell biology of the impaired proliferation of T cells from elderly humans. In: Goidl EA, ed. *Ageing and the immune response*. New York, Marcel Dekker Inc., 1987:67–80.

98. Gottesman SRS. Changes in T-cell-mediated immunity with age: an update. *Review of Biological Research on Ageing*, 1987, **3**:95–127.

99. Chopra RK. Mechanisms of impaired T-cell function in the elderly. *Review of Biological Research on Ageing*, 1990, **4**:83–104.

100. Makinodan T. Patterns of age-related immunologic changes. *Nutrition Reviews*, 1995, **53**:S27–S31.

101. Miller RA et al. Early activation defects in T lymphocytes from aged mice. *Immunology Review*, 1997, **160**:79–90.

102. Weksler ME. Immune senescence: Deficiency or dysregulation? *Nutrition Reviews*, 1995, **53**:S3–S7.

103. Wade AW, Szewczuk MR. Changes in the mucosal-associated B-cell response with age. In: Goidl EA, ed. *Ageing and the immune response.* New York, Marcel Dekker Inc., 1987, 95–121.

104. Nagel JE, Proust JJ. Age-related changes in humoral immunity, complement, and polymorphonuclear leukocyte function. *Review of Biological Research on Ageing,* Journal of Immunology, 1987, **3**:147–159.

105. Ennist DL. Humoral immunosenescense: an update. *Review of Biological Research on Ageing,* 1990, **4**:105–120.

106. Ernst DN, Weigle O, Hobbs MV. Ageing and lymphokine gene expression by T-cell subsets. *Nutrition Reviews,* 1995, **53**:S18–S25.

107. Beharka AA et al. Increased prostaglandin production by murine macrophages contributes to the age-associated decrease in T-cell function. *FASEB Journal,* 1996, **9**:A754.

108. Hayek MG et al. Age differences in eicosanoid production of mouse splenocytes: Effects on mitogen-induced T-cell proliferation. *Journal of Gerontology,* 1994, **49**:B197–B207.

109. Bender BS. Natural killer cells in senescence: analysis of phenotypes and function. *Review of Biological Research,* 1987, **3**:129–138.

110. Bloom ET. Natural killer cells, lymphokine-associated killer cells, and cytolytic T lymphocytes: compartmentalization of age-related changes in cytolytic lymphocytes? *Journal of Gerontology,* 1994, **49**:B85–B92.

111. Krishnaraj R, Blandford G. Age-associated alterations in human natural killer cells: Increased activity as per conventional and kinetic analysis. *Clinical Immunology and Immunopathology,* 1987, **45**:268–285.

112. Chandra S, Chandra RK. Nutrition, immune response and outcome. *Programme for Food Nutrition Science,* 1986, **10**:1–64.

113. Meydani SN. Dietary modulation of the immune response in the aged. *Age,* 1991, **14**:108–115.

114. Meydani SN. Micronutrients and immune function in the elderly. In: Bendich A, Chandra RK, eds. Micronutrients and Immune Functions. New York, *Annals of the New York Academy of Sciences,* 1990:196–207.

115. Chandra RK, Puri S. Nutritional support improves antibody response to influenza virus vaccine in the elderly. *British Medical Journal of Clinical Research Education,* 1985, **291**:705–706.

116. Lesourd BM. Protein undernutrition as the major cause of decreased immune function in the elderly: Clinical and functional implications. *Nutrition Reviews,* 1995, **53**:S86–S94.

117. Ligthart GJ et al. Admission criteria for immunogerontological studies in man: the SENIEUR protocol. *Mechanisms of Ageing and Development,* 1984, **28**:47–55.

118. Meydani SN et al. Oral (n-3) fatty acid supplementation suppresses cytokine production and lymphocyte proliferation: Comparison between young and older women. *Journal of Nutrition,* 1991, **121**:547–555.

119. Meydani SN et al. Immunologic effects of National Cholesterol Education Panel (NCEP) Step-2 diets with and without fish-derived n-3 fatty acid enrichment. *Journal of Clinical Investigation,* 1993, **92**:105–113.

120. Wu D et al. Immunological effects of marine- and plant-derived (n-3) polyunsaturated fatty acids in non-human primates. *American Journal of Clinical Nutrition,* 1996, **63**:273–280.

121. Talbott MC, Miller LK, Kerkvliet N. Pyridoxine supplementation: effect of lymphocyte response in elderly persons. *American Journal of Clinical Nutrition*, 1987, **46**:569–664.

122. Meydani SN et al. Vitamin B6 deficiency impairs interleuken-2 production and lymphocyte proliferation of older adults. *American Journal of Clinical Nutrition*, 1991, **53**:1275–1280.

123. Meydani SN et al. Vitamin E supplementation enhances cell-mediated immunity in healthy elderly subjects. *American Journal of Clinical Nutrition*, 1990, **52**:557–563.

124. Meydani SN et al. Vitamin E supplementation enhances in vivo immune response in healthy elderly subjects: A randomized controlled trial. *Journal of the American Medical Association*, 1997, **277**:1380–1386.

125. Hayek MG et al. Vitamin E supplementation decreases lung virus titres in mice infected with influenza. *Journal of Infectious Diseases*, 1997, **176**:273–276.

126. Han SN et al. Vitamin E supplementation increases T helper 1 cytokine production in old mice infected with influenza virus. *Immunology*, 2000, **100**:487–493.

127. Santos MS et al. Short- and long-term beta-carotene supplementation do not influence T Cell-mediated immunity in healthy elderly. *American Journal of Clinical Nutrition*, 1997, **66**:917–924.

128. Santos MS et al. Natural killer cell activity in elderly men is enhanced by Fl-carotene supplementation. *American Journal of Clinical Nutrition*, 1996, **64**:772–777.

129. Meydani SN et al. Safety assessment of long-term vitamin E supplementation in healthy elderly. *American Journal of Clinical Nutrition*, 1998, **68**:311–318.

130. Kiremidjian-Schumacher L, Roy M. Selenium and immune function. *Zeitschrift fur Ernahrungswissenschaft [Journal of Nutritional Sciences]*, 1998, **37**:50–56.

131. Peretz A et al. Lymphocyte response is enhanced by supplementation of elderly subjects with selenium-enriched yeast. *American Journal of Clinical Nutrition*, 1991, **53**:1323–1328.

132. Meydani SN. Micronutrients and immune function in the elderly. *Annals of the New York Academy of Sciences*, 1990, **587**:196–207.

133. Bogden JD et al. Effects of one year of supplementation with zinc and other micronutrients on cellular immunity in the elderly. *Journal of the American College of Nutrition*, 1990, **9**:214–225.

134. Bogden JD et al. Daily micronutrient supplements enhance delayed-hypersensitivity skin test responses in older people. *American Journal of Clinical Nutrition*, 1994, **60**:437–447.

135. Chandra RK. Effect of vitamin and trace-element supplementation on immune responses and infectious disease in elderly subjects. *Lancet*, 1992, **340**:1124–1127.

136. Penn ND et al. The effect of dietary supplementation with vitamins A, C, and E on cell-mediated immune function in elderly long-stay patients: A randomized, controlled trial. *Age and Ageing*, 1991, **20**:169–174.

137. Buzina-Suboticanec K et al. Ageing, nutritional status, and immune response. *International Journal for Vitamin and Nutrition Research*, 1998, **68**:133–141.

138. Pike J, Chandra RK. Effect of vitamin and trace element supplementation on immune indices in healthy elderly. *International Journal for Vitamin and Nutrition Research*, 1995, **65**:117–121.

139. McKeith IG et al. Consensus guidelines for the clinical and pathologic diagnosis of dementia with Lewy bodies (DLB): report of the consortium on DLB international workshop. *Neurology*, 1996, **47**:1113–1124.

140. Brun A. Frontal lobe degeneration of non-Alzheimer type revisited. *Dementia*, 1993, **4**:126–131.

141. Skoog I. Risk factors for vascular dementia: a review. *Dementia*, 1994, **5**:137–144.

142. Hofman A et al. Atherosclerosis, apolipoprotein E, and prevalence of dementia and Alzheimer's disease in the Rotterdam Study. *Lancet*, 1997, **349**:151–154.

143. Rovner BW et al. Depression and Alzheimer's disease. *American Journal of Psychiatry*, 1989, **146**:350–353.

144. Reifler BV. Diagnosing Alzheimer's disease in the presence of mixed cognitive and affective symptoms. *International Psychogeriatrics*, 1997, **1**:59–64.

145. Braunwald E. Shattuck Lecture. Cardiovascular medicine at the turn of the millennium: triumphs, concerns, and opportunities. *New England Journal of Medicine*, 1997, **337**:1360–1369.

146. Stähelin HB. Antioxidants and atherosclerosis. In: Guesry P, Hennerici H, Sitzer G, eds. *Nutrition and stroke*. Nestlé Nutrition Workshop Series, Supplement. Philadelphia, Lippincott-Raven, 1997:75-86.

147. Gale CR, Martin CN, Cooper C. Cognitive impairment and mortality in a cohort of elderly people. *British Medical Journal*, 1996, **312**:608–611.

148. Lai SM et al. A multifactorial analysis of risk factors for recurrence of ischemic stroke. *Stroke*, 1994, **25**:958–962.

149. Yoshitake T et al. Incidence and risk factors of vascular dementia and Alzheimer's disease in a defined elderly Japanese population: the Hisayama Study. *Neurology*, 1995, **45**:1161–1168.

150. Rosenberg IH, Miller JW. Nutritional factors in physical and cognitive functions of elderly people. *American Journal of Clinical Nutrition*, 1992, **55**:1237S–1243S.

151. Seshadri S et al. Plasma homocysteine as a risk factor for dementia and Alzheimer's disease. *New England Journal of Medicine*, 2002, **346**:476–483.

152. Magistretti PJ, Pellerin L. Regulation by neurotransmitters of glial energy metabolism. *Advances in Experimental Medicine and Biology*, 1997, **429**:137–143.

153. Wurtman RJ, O'Rourke D, Wurtman JJ. Nutrient imbalances in depressive disorders. Possible brain mechanisms. *Annals of the New York Academy of Sciences*, 1989, **575**:75–82, discussion 82–5.

154. Smith KA, Fairburn CG, Cowen PJ. Relapse of depression after rapid depletion of tryptophan. *Lancet*, 1997, **349**:915–919.

155. Alpert JE, Fava M. Nutrition and depression: the role of folate. *Nutrition Reviews*, 1997, **55**:145–149.

156. Goodwin JS, Goodwin JM, Garry PJ. Association between nutritional status and cognitive functioning in a healthy elderly population. *Journal of the American Medical Association*, 1982, **249**:2917–2921.

157. Chome J et al. Effects of suboptimal vitamin status on behaviour. *Bibliotheca Nutritio et Dieta* [Nutrition and Diet Library] (Switzerland), 1986:94–103.

158. Wahlin A et al. Effects of serum vitamin B12 and folate status on episodic memory performance in very old age: a population-based study. *Psychology and Aging*, 1996, **11**:487–496.

159. Perrig WJ, Perrig P, Stähelin HB. The relation between antioxidants and memory performance in the old and very old. *Journal of the American Geriatrics Society*, 1997, **45**:718–724.

160. Widmer LK et al. *Venen-, Arterienkrankheiten, koronare Herzkrankheit bei Berufstaetigen ("Basler Studie")* [Diseases of the veins and arteries and coronary heart disease among the employed ("Basel Study")]. Bern, Hans Huber, 1981.

161. Jama JW et al. Dietary antioxidants and cognitive function in a population-based sample of older persons. The Rotterdam Study. *American Journal of Epidemiology*, 1996, **144**:275–280.

162. Haller J et al. Mental health: minimental state examination and geriatric depression score of elderly Europeans in the SENECA study of 1993. *European Journal of Clinical Nutrition*, 1996, **50**(Suppl. 2):S112-S–116.

163. de Rijk M et al. Dietary antioxidants and Parkinson disease. The Rotterdam Study. *Archives of Neurology*, 1997, **54**:762–765.

164. Meador K et al. Preliminary findings of high-dose thiamine in dementia of Alzheimer's type. *Journal of Geriatric Psychiatry and Neurology*, 1993, **6**:222–229.

165. Fahn S. A pilot trial of high-dose alpha-tocopherol and ascorbate in early Parkinson's disease. *Annals of Neurology*, 1992, **32**:128–132.

166. Fahn S, Cohen G. The oxidant stress hypothesis in Parkinson's disease: evidence supporting it. *Annals of Neurology*, 1992, **32**:804–812.

167. Sano M et al. A controlled trial of selegiline, alpha-tocopherol, or both as treatment for Alzheimer's disease. The Alzheimer's Disease Cooperative Study. *New England Journal of Medicine*, 1997, **336**:1216–1222.

168. Cuajungco MP, Lees GJ. Zinc metabolism in the brain: relevance to human neurodegenerative disorders. *Neurobiology of Disease*, 1997, **4**:137–169.

169. Evans W. What is sarcopenia? *Journal of Gerontology*, 1995, **50**:5–8.

170. Bassey EJ et al. Leg extensor power and functional performance in very old men and women. *Clinical Science*, 1992, **82**:321–327.

171. Meredith CN et al. Body composition and aerobic capacity in young and middle-aged endurance-trained men. *Medicine and Science in Sports and Exercise*, 1987, **19**:557–563.

172. Roberts SB et al. What are the dietary energy needs of elderly adults? *International Journal of Obesity*, 1992, **16**:969–976.

173. Laurent-Winter C, Schnohr P, Saltin B. Function, morphology and protein expression of ageing skeletal muscle: a cross-sectional study of elderly men with different training backgrounds. *Acta Physiologica Scandinavica*, 1990, **140**:41–54.

174. Klitgaard H et al. Ageing alters the myosin heavy chain composition of single fibres from human skeletal muscle. *Acta Physiologica Scandinavica*, 1990, **140**:55–62.

175. Meredith CN et al. Peripheral effects of endurance training in young and old subjects. *Journal of Applied Physiology*, 1989, **66**:2844–2849.

176. Seals DR et al. Endurance training in older men and women. I. Cardiovascular responses to exercise. *Journal of Applied Physiology*, 1984, **57**:1024–1029.

177. Spina RJ et al. Differences in cardiovascular adaptation to endurance exercise training between older men and women. *Journal of Applied Physiology*, 1993, **75**:849–855.

178. Davidson MB. The effect of ageing on carbohydrate metabolism. A review of the English literature and a practical approach to the diagnosis of Diabetes Mellitus in the elderly. *Metabolism*, 1979, **28**:688–705.

179. Hadden WC, Harris MI. Prevalence of diagnosed diabetes, undiagnosed diabetes, and impaired glucose tolerance in adults 20–74 years of age: United States, 1976-1980. In: *DHHS PHS Publication No. 87–1687*. Washington, DC, US Government Printing Office, 1987.

180. Shimokata H et al. Age as independent determinant of glucose tolerance. *Diabetes*, 1991, **40**:44–51.

181. Borkan GA, Hultz DE, Gerzoff AF. Age changes in body composition revealed by computed tomography. *Journal of Gerontology*, 1983, **38**:673–677.

182. Stolk RP et al. Retinopathy, glucose and insulin in an elderly population: The Rotterdam study. *Diabetes*, 1995, **44**:11–15.

183. Zavaroni I et al. Effect of age and environmental factors on glucose tolerance and insulin secretion in a worker population. *Journal of the American Geriatric Society*, 1986, **34**:271–275.

184. Seals DR et al. Effects of endurance training on glucose tolerance and plasma lipid levels in older men and women. *Journal of the American Medical Association*, 1984, **252**:645–649.

185. Kirwan JP et al. Endurance exercise training reduces glucose-stimulated insulin levels in 60- to 70-year-old men and women. *Journal of Gerontology*, 1993, **48**:M84–M90.

186. Hughes VA et al. Exercise increases muscle GLUT 4 levels and insulin action in subjects with impaired glucose tolerance. *American Journal of Physiology*, 1993, **264**:E855–E862.

187. Marshall JA, Hamman RF, Baxter J. High-fat, low-carbohydrate diet and the etiology of non-insulin-dependent diabetes mellitus: the San Luis Valley Diabetes Study. *American Journal of Epidemiology*, 1991, **134**:590–603.

188. Feskens EJM, Kromhout D. Cardiovascular risk factors and the 25-year incidence of diabetes mellitus in middle-aged men. *American Journal of Epidemiology*, 1989, **130**: 1101–1108.

189. Lundgren J et al. Dietary habits and incidence of noninsulin-dependent diabetes mellitus in a population study of women in Gothenburg, Sweden. *American Journal of Clinical Nutrition*, 1989, **52**:708–712.

190. Borkman M et al. Comparison of the effects on insulin sensitivity of high carbohydrate and high-fat diets in normal subjects. *Journal of Clinical Endocrinology*, 1991, **72**:432–437.

191. Garg A, Grundy SM, Unger RH. Comparison of effects of high and low carbohydrate diets on plasma lipoprotein and insulin sensitivity in patients with mild NIDDM. *Diabetes*, 1992, **41**:1278–1285.

192. Hughes VA et al. Long-term effects of a high carbohydrate diet and exercise on insulin action in older subjects with impaired glucose tolerance. *American Journal of Clinical Nutrition*, 1995, **62**:426–433.

193. Schaefer EJ et al. Body weight and low-density lipoprotein cholesterol changes after consumption of a low-fat ad libitum diet. *Journal of the American Medical Association*, 1995, **274**:1450–1455.

194. Helmrich SP et al. Physical activity and reduced occurrence of non-insulin-dependent diabetes mellitus. *New England Journal of Medicine*, 1991, **325**:147–152.

195. Bogardus C et al. Effects of physical training and diet therapy on carbohydrate metabolism in patients with glucose intolerance and non-insulin-dependent diabetes mellitus. *Diabetes*, 1984, **33**:311–318.

196. Phinney SD et al. Effects of aerobic exercise on energy expenditure and nitrogen balance during very low calorie dieting. *Metabolism*, 1988, **37**:758–765.

197. Heymsfield SB et al. Rate of weight loss during underfeeding: relation to level of physical activity. *Metabolism*, 1989, **38**:215–223.

198. Goran MI, Poehlman ET. Endurance training does not enhance total energy expenditure in healthy elderly persons. *American Journal of Physiology*, 1992, **263**:E950–E957.

199. Withers RT et al. Energy metabolism in sedentary and active 49- to 70-year-old women. *Journal of Applied Physiology*, 1998, **84**:1333–1340.

200. Ballor DL et al. Resistance weight training during caloric restriction enhances lean body weight maintenance. *American Journal of Clinical Nutrition*, 1988, **47**:19–25.

201. Pavlou, KN et al. Effects of dieting and exercise on lean body mass, oxygen uptake, and strength. *Medicine and Science in Sports and Exercise*, 1985, **17**:466–471.

202. Evans WJ, Cannon JG. The metabolic effects of exercise-induced muscle damage. In: Holloszy JO, ed. *Exercise and Sport Sciences Reviews*. Baltimore, Williams & Wilkins, **199**:99–126.

203. Nelson ME et al. Effects of high-intensity strength training on multiple risk factors for osteoporotic fractures. *Journal of the American Medical Association*, 1994, **272**:1909–1914.

204. Frontera WR et al. Strength training and determinants of VO2max in older men. *Journal of Applied Physiology*, 1990, **68**:329–333.

205. Fleg JL, Lakatta EG. Role of muscle loss in the age-associated reduction in VO2max. *Journal of Applied Physiology*, 1988, **65**:1147–1151.

206. Fiatarone MA et al. High-intensity strength training in nonagenarians. Effects on skeletal muscle. *Journal of the American Medical Association*, 1990, **263**:3029–3034.

207. Fiatarone MA et al. Exercise training and nutritional supplementation for physical frailty in very elderly people. *New England Journal of Medicine*, 1994, **330**:1769–1775.

208. Sahyoun N. Nutrient intake by the NSS elderly population. In: Hartz SC, Russell RM, Rosenberg IH, eds. *Nutrition in the elderly: The Boston Nutritional Status Survey*. London, Smith-Gordon and Company, 1992.

209. Launer LJ et al. Body mass index, weight change, and risk of mobility disability in middle-aged and older women. *Journal of the American Medical Association*, 1994, **271**:1093–1098.

210. Metropolitan Life Insurance Company. *The 1979 build study*. Chicago, Society of Actuaries and Association of Life Insurance Medical Directors of America, 1980.

211. Micozzi MS, Harris TM. Age variations in the relation of body mass index to estimates of body fat and muscle mass. *American Journal of Physiology and Anthropology*, 1990, **81**:375–379.

212. Roubenoff R, Dallal GE, Wilson PWF. Predicting body fat: the body mass index vs. estimation by bioelectrical impedance. *American Journal of Public Health*, 1995, **85**:726–728.

213. Smalley KJ et al. Reassessment of body mass indices. *American Journal of Clinical Nutrition*, 1990, **52**:405–408.

214. Kehayias JJ et al. Total body potassium and body fat: relevance to ageing. *American Journal of Clinical Nutrition*, 1997, **66**:904–910.

215. Roubenoff R, Kehayias JJ. The meaning and measurement of lean body mass. *Nutrition Reviews*, 1991, **46**:163–175.

216. Roubenoff R et al. Bioelectrical impedance equations in ambulatory elderly Caucasians. *Journal of Gerontology* 1997, **52**:M129–M136.

217. Roubenoff R. Applications of bioelectrical impedance analysis for body composition to epidemiologic studies. *American Journal of Clinical Nutrition*, 1996, **64**:459S–462S.

218. Guralnick J et al. A short physical performance battery assessing lower extremity function. *Journal of Gerontology*, 1994, **49**:M85–M94.

219. Heikkinen E, Waters WE, Brzezinski ZJ, eds. *The elderly in eleven countries—a sociomedical survey*. Copenhagen, World Health Organization, Regional Office for Europe, Public Health in Europe Series, No. 21, 1983.

220. Katz S, Downs TO, Cash HR. Progression in the development of the index ADL. *The Gerontologist*, 1970, **1**:20–30.

221. *Preparation and Use of Food-Based Dietary Guidelines. Report of a joint FAO/WHO consultation*. Geneva, World Health Organization, 1996 (WHO Technical Report Series, No. 880).

222. Roberts SR, Young VR. Ageing and energy metabolism. *Proceedings of the XVth Congress of the International Association of Gerontology.* Budapest, Hungary. Monduzzi S.p.A., Bologna, ed, 1993:269–376.

223. Saltzman E, Roberts SB. Effects of energy imbalance on energy expenditure and respiratory quotient in young and older men: a summary of data from two metabolic studies. *Aging*, 1996, **8**:370–378.

224. Knox TA et al. Calcium absorption in elderly subjects on high- and low-fibre diets: effects of gastric acidity. *American Journal of Clinical Nutrition*, 1991, **53**:1480–1486.

225. Prince RL et al. Prevention of postmenopausal osteoporosis. A comparative study of exercise, calcium supplementation, and hormone replacement therapy. *New England Journal of Medicine*, 1991, **325**:1189–1195.

226. Polley KJ et al. Effect of calcium supplementation on forearm bone mineral content in postmenopausal women: a prospective sequential controlled trial. *Journal of Nutrition*, 1987, **117**:1929–1935.

227. Dawson-Hughes B et al. A Controlled trial of the effect of calcium supplementation on bone density in postmenopausal women. *New England Journal of Medicine*, 1990, **323**:878–883.

228. Bunker VW et al. Assessment of zinc and copper status of healthy elderly people using metabolic balance studies and measurement of leukocyte concentrations. *American Journal of Clinical Nutrition*, 1984, **40**:1096–1102.

229. *Trace elements in human nutrition.* Geneva, World Health Organization, 1996.

230. Wood RJ, Suter PM, Russell RM. Mineral requirements of elderly people. *American Journal of Clinical Nutrition*, 1995, **62**:493–505.

231. Mertz W et al. Trace elements in the elderly. Metabolism requirements, and recommendations for intakes. In: Munro HM, Danfoard DE, eds. *Nutrition, ageing and the elderly.* Vol. 6. New York, Plenum Press, 1989:195–244.

232. Abraham AS, Brooks BA, Eylath U. The effects of chromium supplementation on serum glucose and lipids in patients with and without non-insulin-dependent diabetes. *Metabolism*, 1992, **41**:768–771.

233. Offenbacher EG et al. Metabolic chromium balances in men. *American Journal of Clinical Nutrition*, 1986, **44**:77–82.

234. *Fats and oils in human nutrition. Report of a joint FAO/WHO expert consultation.* Rome, Food and Agriculture Organization of the United Nations (FAO Food and Nutrition Paper No. 57, 1994).

235. Jagerstad M, Westesson AK. Folate. *Scandinavian Journal of Gastroenterology*, 1979, **14** (Suppl. 53):196–202.

236. Rosenberg IH. Folate, In: Hartz SC, Rosenberg IH, Russell RM, eds. *Nutrition in the elderly.* The Boston Nutritional Status Survey. London, Smith-Gordon & Co Ltd, 1992:135–139.

237. Selhub J et al. Vitamin status and intake as primary determinants of homocysteinemia in an elderly population. *Journal of the American Medical Association*, 1993, **270**: 2693–2698.

238. Yip R, Dallman PR. The roles of inflammation and iron deficiency as causes of anaemia. *American Journal of Clinical Nutrition*, 1988, **48**:1295–1300.

239. Milman N, Andersen HC, Pedersen NS. Serum ferritin and iron status in "healthy" elderly subjects. *Scandinavian Journal of Clinical Laboratory Investigation*, 1986, **46**: 19–26.

240. Campbell WW, Ewans WJ. Protein requirements of elderly people. *European Journal of Clinical Nutrition*, 1985, **50**:S180–S185.

241. Castaneda C et al. Elderly women accommodate to a low-protein diet with losses of body cell mass, muscle function, and immune response. *American Journal of Clinical Nutrition*, 1995, **62**:30–39.

242. Boisvert WA, Russell RM. Riboflavin requirement of healthy elderly humans and its relationship to macronutrient composition of the diet. *Journal of Nutrition*, 1993, **123**:915–925.

243. Horwitt MK et al. Correlation of urinary excretion with dietary intake and symptoms of riboflavinosis. *Journal of Nutrition*, 1950, **41**:247–264.

244. Bunker VW et al. Selenium balance studies in apparently healthy and housebound elderly people eating self-selected diets. *British Journal of Nutrition*, 1988, **59**:171–180.

245. Carmel R et al. Food cobalamin malabsorption occurs frequently in patients with unexplained low serum cobalamin levels. *Archives of Internal Medicine*, 1988, **148**:1715–1719.

246. Krasinski SD et al. Fundic atrophic gastritis in an elderly population. Effect on hemoglobin and several serum nutritional indicators. *Journal of the American Geriatrics Society*, 1986, **34**:800–806.

247. Hurwitz A et al. Gastric acidity in older adults. *Journal of the American Medical Association*, 1997, **278**:659–662.

248. Asaka M et al. What role does *Helicobactor pylori* play in gastric cancer? *Gastroenterology*, 1997, **113**:556–560.

249. Suter PM et al. Reversal of protein-bound vitamin B12 malabsorption with antibiotics in atrophic gastritis. *Gastroenterology*, 1991, **101**:1039–1045.

250. Institute of Medicine. *Dietary Reference Intakes for thiamin, riboflavin, niacin, vitamin B6, folate, vitamin B12, pantothenic acid, biotin and choline*. Washington, DC, National Academy Press, 1998,.

251. Omenn GS et al. Effects of a combination of beta-carotene and vitamin A on lung cancer and cardiovascular disease. *New England Journal of Medicine*, 1996, **334**:1150–1155.

252. Hennekens CH et al. Lack of effect of long-term supplementation with beta-carotene on the incidence of malignant neoplasms and cardiovascular disease. *New England Journal of Medicine*, 1996, **334**:1145–1149.

253. Krasinski SD et al. Relationship of vitamin A and vitamin E intake to fasting plasma retinol, retinol-binding protein, retinyl esters, carotene, alpha-tocopherol, and cholesterol among elderly people and young adults: increased plasma retinyl esters among vitamin A-supplement users. *American Journal of Clinical Nutrition*, 1989, **49**:112–120.

254. Euronut-SENECA Investigators. Intake of vitamins and minerals. *European Journal of Clinical Nutrition*, 1991, **45** (Suppl.):121–138.

255. Haller J et al. Nutritional status: blood vitamins A, E, B6, B12, folic acid and carotene. *European Journal of Clinical Nutrition*, 1991, **45** (Suppl. 3):63–82.

256. Blanchard J et al. Vitamin C disposition in young and elderly men. *American Journal of Clinical Nutrition*, 1990, **51**:837–845.

257. Blanchard J. Depletion and repletion kinetics of vitamin C in humans. *Journal of Nutrition*, 1990, **121**:170–176.

258. VanderJagt DJ, Garry PJ, Bhagavan HN. Ascorbic acid intake and plasma levels in healthy elderly people. *American Journal of Clinical Nutrition*, 1987, **46**:290–294.

259. Frei B. Ascorbic acid protects lipids in human plasma and low-density lipoprotein against oxidative damage. *American Journal of Clinical Nutrition*, 1991, **54**:S1113–S1118.

260. Jialal I, Vega GL, Grundy SM. Physiologic levels of ascorbate inhibit the oxidative modification of low density lipoprotein. *Atherosclerosis*, 1990, **82**:185–191.

261. Nyyssonen K et al. Vitamin C deficiency and risk of myocardial infarction: prospective population study of men from eastern Finland. *British Medical Journal*, 1997, **314**: 634–638.

262. Ferland G, Sadowski JA, O'Brien ME. Dietary induced subclinical vitamin K deficiency in normal human subjects. *Journal of Clinical Investigations*, 1993, **91**:1761–1768.

263. Dawson-Hughes B et al. Effect of vitamin D supplementation on wintertime overall bone loss in healthy postmenopausal women. *Annals of Internal Medicine*, 1991, **115**: 505–512.

264. Meydani SN et al. Vitamin E supplementation and in vivo immune response in healthy elderly subjects. A randomized controlled trial. *Journal of the American Medical Association*, 1997, **277**:1380–1386.

265. Jacques PF et al. Antioxidant status in persons with and without senile cataract. *Archives of Ophthalmology*, 1988, **106**:337–340.

266. Knekt P et al. Vitamin E and cancer prevention. *American Journal of Clinical Nutrition*, 1991, **53**:S283–S286.

267. Sano M et al. A controlled trial of selegiline, alpha-tocopherol, or both as treatment for Alzheimer's disease. *New England Journal of Medicine*, 1997, **336**:1216–1222.

268. Stephens NG et al. Randomized control trial of vitamin E in patients with coronary diseases: Cambridge Heart Antioxidant Study (CHAOS). *Lancet*, 1996, **347**:781–786.

269. Rapola JM et al. Effect of vitamin E and beta carotene on the incidence of angina pectoris. A randomized, double-blind, controlled trial. *Journal of the American Medical Association*, 1996, **275**:693–698.

270. Bach AU et al. Assessment of vitamin K status in human subjects administered a "minidose" warfarin. *American Journal of Clinical Nutrition*, 1996, **64**:894–902.

271. Booth SSL et al. Relationship between dietary intakes and fasting plasma concentrations of fat-soluble vitamins in humans. *Journal of Nutrition*, 1997, **127**:587–592.

Ageing and Health
Report by the WHO Secretariat[1]

At its fifty-fourth session in 2000, the United Nations General Assembly decided to convene a second world assembly on ageing in order to review the outcome of the first World Assembly on Ageing (Vienna 1982). WHO participated actively in all the preparatory meetings. As its principal technical contribution to the Second World Assembly on Ageing (Madrid, 8 to 12 April 2002), WHO introduced its policy framework on active ageing,[2] which focuses on such areas as:

- preventing and reducing the burden of disabilities, chronic disease and premature mortality;

- reducing the risk factors associated with noncommunicable diseases and functional decline as individuals age, while increasing factors that protect health;

- enacting policies and strategies that provide a continuum of care for people with chronic illness or disabilities;

- providing training and education to formal and informal carers;

- ensuring the protection, safety and dignity of ageing individuals;

- enabling people as they age to maintain their contribution to economic development, to activity in the formal and informal sectors, and to their communities and families.

The Assembly adopted two documents: the Political Declaration and the International Plan of Action on Ageing 2002.

In the **Political Declaration**,[3] governments expressed their commitment to act at national and international levels on three priority directions: older persons and development; advancing health and well-being into old age; and ensuring enabling and supportive environments. The Declaration recognizes that persons, as they age, should enjoy a life of fulfilment, health, security and active participation in the economic, social, cultural and political life of their societies. It acknowledges that new opportunities exist to enable men and women to reach old age in better

---

[1] Adapted from documents A55/17 and A55/17 Add.1. Fifty-fifth World Health Assembly, Geneva, World Health Organization, 13–18 May 2002, http://www.who.int/gb/.

[2] http://www.who.int/hpr/ageing/ActiveAgeingPolicyFrame.pdf

[3] http://www.un.org/esa/socdev/ageing/waa/

health, and that empowerment and promotion of full participation in society are essential elements for active ageing. It reaffirms that the attainment of the highest possible level of health is a most important social goal, whose realization requires action by many social and economic sectors in addition to that of health. While assigning the primary responsibility to provide leadership on ageing matters to governments, it underlines the important role of the United Nations system in providing support to governments in implementation and follow-up of the International Plan of Action on Ageing.

The **International Plan of Action on Ageing 2002**[1] briefly analyses the three priority areas and sets out objectives and actions to be pursued. It deals, among other matters, with advancing health and well-being into old age. Paragraphs 57 to 66 take a **life course perspective** in health promotion and disease prevention. Specific objectives and actions address the cumulative effects of certain risk factors, such as tobacco use, alcohol consumption, inadequate access to food and clean water, and unhealthy nutrition leading to disease and dependency in later life.

Paragraphs 67 to 73 are devoted to providing **universal and equal access** to health care services for older persons. The ultimate goal is to provide a continuum of care, ranging from health promotion and disease prevention to the provision of primary health care, acute care, chronic care, rehabilitation services, long-term care, and palliative care for older persons suffering incurable illnesses. The responsibility of governments for setting and monitoring standards of health care and care provision is stressed. Although partnerships among government, civil society and the private sector are valuable, the Plan recognizes that services provided by the family and community cannot substitute for an effective public health system.

Paragraphs 74 to 77 address the impact of HIV/AIDS on older persons, including the key role they play as primary care givers for people living with HIV/AIDS and their families, notably orphaned children.

The urgent need to widen opportunities in the field of **geriatrics and gerontology** for all health professionals as well as informal carers is referred to in paragraphs 78 and 79. Paragraphs 80 and 81 provide guidance for actions for the development of **comprehensive mental health care services**, ranging from prevention, early diagnosis and intervention to provision of treatment and the management of mental health problems among older persons.

Paragraphs 82 to 84 deal with the **maintenance of maximum functional capacity** throughout the life course and the promotion of the full participation of older persons with disabilities in society. With respect to disabilities, the especially vulnerable situation of older women is highlighted. The importance of establishing age-friendly standards and environments is stressed as a means of preventing the onset and the worsening of disabilities among older persons. Similar interest is

---

[1] http://www.un.org/esa/socdev/ageing/waa/

expressed in paragraphs 87 to 92, with particular reference to barrier-free and accessible housing and transportation systems.

An area not previously addressed in a United Nations action plan is that of **neglect, abuse and violence** against older people (paragraphs 98 to 101). Acknowledging that such ill-treatment takes many forms—physical, psychological, emotional and financial—action is recommended in the areas of education, awareness-raising, and the creation of health and social support services. In particular, the need to address the gender dimensions of abuse of older people is emphasized.

Governments have the primary responsibility for implementing the recommendations of the Plan of Action. National efforts are to be complemented and enhanced through coordinated actions at international level. The United Nations system, through its specialized agencies, will be expected to develop strategies for implementation in the areas of their respective mandates. The Plan singled out training and capacity-building in developing countries as areas needing the support of the international development agencies. Implementation of the Plan is to be set in the context of the objectives of the Millennium Declaration and follow-up of major United Nations conferences.

More specifically, the Plan recommends that the focal points that were set up within the organizations of the United Nations system in preparation for the Assembly should be maintained and strengthened in order to enhance their institution's capacity to implement the Plan.

List of participants
World Health Organization/Tufts University Consultation on Nutritional Guidelines for the Elderly

USDA Human Nutrition Research Center on Aging at Tufts University, Boston, MA, 26–29 May 1998

Dr Irwin H. Rosenberg, Director, United States Department of Agriculture (USDA) Human Nutrition Research Center on Aging, Tufts University, Boston, Massachusetts, USA (Chairman)

Experts

Dr Allen Balsam, Commissioner of Health, Brookline, Massachusetts, USA

Dr Jeffrey Blumberg, USDA Human Nutrition Research Center on Aging, Tufts University

Dr Carmen Castenada, USDA Human Nutrition Research Center on Aging, Tufts University

Dr Vijay Chandra, Director, Centre for Ageing Research, New Delhi, India

Dr J. Grimley Evans, Division of Geriatric Medicine, University of Oxford, Oxford, United Kingdom of Great Britain and Northern Ireland

Dr William J. Evans, Nutrition, Metabolism and Exercise Program, University of Arkansas for Medical Sciences, Little Rock, Arkansas, USA

Dr P.R. Kenya, Faculty of Health Sciences, Moi University, Eldoret, Kenya

Dr Anura V. Kurpad, Department of Physiology and Nutrition Research Centre, St John's Medical College, Bangalore, India

Dr Simin Meydani, USDA Human Nutrition Research Center on Aging, Tufts University

Dr Susan Roberts, USDA Human Nutrition Research Center on Aging, Tufts University

Dr Ronenn Roubenoff, USDA Human Nutrition Research Center on Aging, Tufts University

Dr Robert Russell, USDA Human Nutrition Research Center on Aging, Tufts University

Dr Nevin S. Scrimshaw, Food & Nutrition Programme, United Nations University

Professor H.B. Stähelin, University Geriatric Clinic, Kantonsspital, Basel, Switzerland

Dr Mark Wahlqvist, Monash University, Clayton, Australia

World Health Organization

Mr James Akré, Department of Nutrition for Health and Development (contributing editor)

Dr Ratko Buzina, Department of Nutrition for Health and Development

Dr Graeme Clugston, Director, Department of Nutrition for Health and Development

Ms Irene Hoskins, Ageing and Life Course

Dr Nikolai Khaltaev, Management of Noncommunicable Diseases

Assisting editors

Ms Gabriella Amersbach, Tufts University

Ms Maeve D. McNally, Tufts University

Ms Jo Obelsky, Tufts University

Food-based dietary guidelines for older adults
Healthy ageing and prevention of chronic noncommunicable diseases

ML Wahlqvist,[1] A Kouris-Blazos,[2] G Savige[3]

A3.1 Introduction

Instead of making recommendations about the dietary advice that older persons should receive, this section concentrates on some of their key nutritional problems which should be taken into account when developing country- and cuisine-specific food-based dietary guidelines. Australia, Japan and the USA are used as examples given the number of relevant studies available for these countries. The process by which food-based dietary guidelines should be developed, implemented and monitored is discussed in greater detail elsewhere (*1*).

The nutritional needs of an ageing population require special attention. Energy expenditure declines with age; thus, to achieve energy balance, less energy needs to be consumed. This reduction in energy intake can have an adverse effect on the nutritional status of older people unless high nutritional quality foods are eaten, such as fish, lean meat, eggs, low-fat dairy products, whole-grain cereals, seeds, nuts, legumes, fruits and vegetables.

Consuming foods that are rich in nutrients and other bioactive components (such as phytochemicals) may also help to protect against major age-related disorders such as immunocompetence and cognitive impairment (*2–3*). However, being free of illness does not necessarily ensure good quality of life as one ages. Mobility, independence, cognitive function, psychological state, and social relations and networks are also very important (*4–8*), and they need to be maintained—in part through good nutrition—well into old age.

A3.2 Is it too late to give dietary advice to older persons?

At age 65 men and women in high-income countries still have a life expectancy of around 15 and 19 years, respectively. The older one becomes, the longer one is likely to live, and thus, by the time men and women reach age 75, life expectancy is still 9 and 11 years, respectively. A common assumption is that changes in lifestyle

---

[1] Professor of Medicine, Monash Medical School, Prahran 3181, Australia; President, International Union of Nutritional Sciences.

[2] Honorary Research Fellow, Asia Pacific Health and Nutrition Centre, Monash Asia Institute, Monash University.

[3] Senior Training Officer, Monash University, FAO Centre of Excellence, Monash Medical School, Alfred Hospital, Prahran 3181, Australia.

to improve health are no longer worthwhile in old age, and that the remaining years are insufficient to reap the benefits of dietary modifications. Yet the prevalence of heart disease, diabetes, hypertension, obesity and arthritis is highest in the older population. Intervention trials demonstrate that there are still worthwhile health advantages for older persons in changing risk factors—e.g. smoking cessation, weight reduction, sodium restriction, saturated fat reduction—and that these changes make later years healthier, more active and less dependent (*9*).

A3.3 **Food-based dietary guidelines**

Most dietary guidelines are based on individual nutrients (fat, alcohol, salt, sugar, calcium and iron) and food groups (e.g. eat more vegetables and cereals, consume less fat). However, food-based dietary guidelines go beyond nutrients and food groups; they include the way foods are produced (agriculture), prepared (cuisine), processed (the food industry) and developed (novel/functional foods). Such guidelines are both practical and user-friendly because they consider traditional foods and dishes and, most importantly, specific cuisines. This paradigm shift is likely to make a significant contribution to human health, to help maintain cultural diversity and to optimize nutritional status in a sustainable environment. The aim of food-based dietary guidelines is to reduce chronic malnutrition, micronutrient malnutrition, and diet-related communicable and noncommunicable diseases (*1, 10*).

National nutrient-based dietary guidelines have met with only moderate success since they fail to include key factors such as traditional foods and dishes, eating patterns, food availability and sustainable food production. Furthermore, providing consumers dietary guidelines that are primarily nutrient focused can have unintended consequences. For example, advice to avoid too much fat can be interpreted as guidance to eliminate *all* sources of dietary fat rather than to choose leaner versions of foods that remain important nutrient sources.

Food-based dietary guidelines provide an opportunity to improve the effectiveness of nutrition education for the general public. They do this by taking into account information concerning both food consumption and nutrient intake and by incorporating this knowledge within a culturally sensitive framework (11). Food-based dietary guidelines allow the principles of nutrition education to be expressed, qualitatively and quantitatively, mostly as foods and culture-specific dishes, thereby making them as practical as possible. Since the guidelines are intended for use by individuals, they can largely avoid using technical terms of nutritional science.

Country- and cuisine-specific food-based dietary guidelines focus directly on diet and disease relationships of particular relevance to individual countries. For example, specific priorities to be addressed through food-based dietary guidelines depend on whether public health concerns relate to dietary insufficiency or excess or, indeed, to a combination of both. They also need to consider social, economic, agricultural and environmental factors affecting food availability and eating patterns, while recognizing that more than one dietary pattern is consistent with health (*10*).

Food-based dietary guidelines encourage the maintenance of healthy traditional dishes and cooking practices. They are sensitive to local agriculture and whether it can support the guidance provided. Such guidelines can also take into account the positive and negative nutritional effects that follow changes in dietary patterns, e.g. post-migration changes to traditional diets and acculturation to mainstream diets. Food-based dietary guidelines can be structured to enable a population to meet recommended dietary intakes of all known essential nutrients, especially where nutrient deficiency has been linked to diet-related public health problems, e.g. essential fatty acids or folic acid and cardiovascular disease (*12, 13*).

Furthermore, diet-related disorders are dependent not only on increased intakes of detrimental foods, e.g. fatty meat, full-fat dairy products, but also on reduced intakes of protective foods such as fish (*14, 15*), fruits and vegetables, and beverages such as tea (*16, 17*). Because the protective-food approach to chronic noncommunicable diseases (CNCD) is poorly developed in nutritional science, the food-based dietary guideline approach has a considerable advantage over the nutrient-based approach. Food variety is probably the best available encapsulation of the food-based dietary guideline approach to reducing detriment to health and enhancing health protection through diet (*18–20*).

In addition to national food-based dietary guidelines, policy-makers and health care professionals can use dietary guidelines expressed in terms of quantitative nutrient and food component recommendations. Government bodies responsible for developing food-based dietary guidelines are encouraged to integrate these messages with other health-related policies, e.g. smoking cessation, increased physical activity and lowered alcohol consumption. To review these issues in practical policy terms, FAO and WHO jointly organized a consultation on the preparation and use of food-based dietary guidelines. The consultation's report provides for a reorientation from nutrients to foods in developing dietary guidelines (10); their implementation is discussed elsewhere (*1*).

A3.4 Selecting a target group for food-based dietary guidelines

Selecting a target group for establishing food-based dietary guidelines will have a major influence on their form and content mode of dissemination. Target groups can be categorized according to three levels (*21*):

- General, e.g. older children and adults.
- Specific, e.g. pregnant/lactating women, infants, preschool children, older persons, vegetarians.

- Patients with certain disorders or diseases, e.g. diarrhoea, atherosclerosis, and liver and renal diseases.

Food-based dietary guidelines need to show that, although serving sizes will vary according to age groups, a family can eat together from a common plate. Foods and snacks eaten alone may have to be targeted. It may be better to have one set of guidelines within which special mention is made of specific age, or otherwise vulnerable, groups, or that deal with their needs via supplementary guidelines. Health professionals can use therapeutic or curative guidelines on a one-to-one basis or for small-group counselling for patients with certain disorders or diseases. If therapeutic or curative guidelines are developed, they probably should not be referred to as dietary guidelines. Another name, for example therapeutic guidelines, would be preferable.

In Australia there are specific dietary guidelines for adults and children, and working groups that deal with aboriginal nutrition and obesity. Dietary guidelines for older persons and pregnant women have also been identified as priority areas. However, Japan is the only country with specific dietary guidelines for older persons (*22*), including the following main recommendations.

Beware of undernutrition; a decrease in weight is a warning sign.

- Make your diet more enjoyable through appropriate cooking; eat a variety of foods and avoid overeating.
- Start with entrees and vegetable dishes; entrees and vegetable dishes are nutritionally more important.
- Eat regularly; take your time to finish each meal; do not skip meals.
- Be active; food tastes better when you are hungry.
- Increase your nutritional knowledge; nutritional knowledge keeps you young and healthy.
- Enjoy your life and enjoy your food; live a full and healthy life.

A3.5 Health concerns covered by food-based dietary guidelines for older adults

As socioeconomic circumstances have improved and effective disease-control programmes have been implemented, survival beyond childhood has increased. The resulting demographic transition (*23*) is characterized by increased life expectancy and a larger proportion of the population moving into the age range where CNCDs became the major cause of ill-health and death. At the same time, there has been an epidemiological transition in diseases due to dietary shifts and a higher prevalence of other risk factors for CNCDs.

A recent report on the global burden of disease (*24*) forecast that deaths from communicable, perinatal, maternal and nutritional conditions will decrease globally by one-third between 1990 and 2020. In contrast, deaths from CNCDs, including heart disease and depression, will *increase* twofold, as will deaths from injuries due to accidents. By 2020, tobacco is expected to cause more premature deaths and disability than any other single factor. These forecasts are conditioned by the rapid ageing of populations in low-income countries. As birth rates fall, the number of adults increases relative to the number of children, and the most common health problems become those of older adults.

Many countries face health risks that are associated with traditional environmental exposures (e.g. poor sanitation), modern agricultural hazards (e.g. pesticide contamination of water and food) and urbanization and industrialization (e.g. CNCDs). While some populations are grappling with problems of undernutrition (e.g. Papua New Guinea, Philippines) still others are beset more by health problems associated with over-nutrition (e.g. Australia, Hong Kong Special Administrative Region of China, New Zealand and Singapore). Countries undergoing nutrition transition are confronted simultaneously by both the old problems of nutrient deficiencies and the new problems of overnutrition (e.g. China, Malaysia, Thailand and China (Province of Taiwan)) (*25*). Currently, dietary guidelines around the world typically tend to focus on specific CNCDs (*26*):

- Obesity (especially abdominal)
- Diabetes (or impaired glucose tolerance)
- Cardiovascular disease
- Certain cancers (lung, breast, colorectal, prostate, pancreas and brain)
- Osteopenia and osteoporosis

A new wave of health problems and diseases requires nutritional analyses and a systematic review of dietary guidelines (*1, 2*); they include:

- Ageing and age-associated frailty
- Protracted menopause with increased longevity in women
- Cognitive impairment and dementia
- Behavioural and psychological disorders (especially in the light of increasing urbanization)
- New infectious diseases
- Environmental diseases (due to chemical residues, atmospheric pollution and damage to the ecosystem)
- Risks and benefits of new foods.

The challenge is to minimize new health problems through environmentally sensitive food-based dietary guidelines, which people themselves understand and control. The quest for new foods to improve health (e.g. in relation to certain

CNCDs) may create new problems where risk-benefit analysis has been inadequate or where consequences are unintended.

There is growing awareness of nutrition's contribution to the major health problems of older persons (*1, 2*), including:

- Protein-energy dysnutrition
- Immune dysfunction
- Macrovascular diseases
- Insulin resistance syndromes
- Renal impairment
- Arthritis
- Osteopenia and fractures
- Neoplastic disease
- Cognitive impairment
- Mood disturbance and depression
- Visual impairment

Several health problems and bodily changes that are typically attributed to the normal ageing process are increasingly recognized as being linked to lifestyle or environmental factors. For example, the decline in lean body mass and the increase in body fat that tend to occur as people age cannot be entirely attributed to the ageing process *per se*. The decline in physical activity with advancing age contributes to a loss of muscle and a decline in basal metabolic rate. Not only is the burden of CNCDs among older persons generally greater than in younger age groups, but associated body compositional disorders, together with loss of lean and bone mass, also contribute to frailty.

A3.5.1 *Compression of morbidity towards the end of life*

Buskirk's review of data on health maintenance and exercise (*27*) supports the assumption that regular exercise blunts many aspects of the psychological decline associated with ageing and improves a sense of well-being and quality of life. Adoption of a healthy physically active lifestyle contributes to a principal health goal for successful ageing, which is to compress morbidity towards the end of life (*28*).

Physical activity among older persons is associated with greater energy intakes, improved nutrient intakes and better quality of life (*29*). Prospective studies show that greater energy intakes balanced with adequate physical activity contribute to decreased cardiovascular disease (*30–32*), total mortality (*33*) and improved life expectancy (*34*). Increasing energy intake runs counter to the disturbing view that restricting energy somehow prolongs life. Rats have been subjected to energy-restricting diets for this purpose, but this approach has no direct application to humans (*35*). Furthermore, energy restriction in older persons may contribute to frailty and loss of lean mass.

A3.5.2 **Frailty and sarcopenia**

Frailty is the most usual descriptor of reduced quality of life and morbidity among older persons; it is more likely to be avoided where physical activity (simple endurance activity such as walking combined with strengthening exercises) and adequate food intake are combined (*36*). Loss of lean mass, accompanied by falls and fractures and proneness to infection (*37, 38*), is the principal nutritional concern for older persons worldwide (*39, 40*). The decline in lean body mass is due largely to a loss in skeletal muscle known as sarcopenia (*41*), whose prevalence, incidence and cause require further study (*42*).

Protein requirements of older people may be higher than currently recommended levels (0.75 g protein/kg per day). An estimated mean protein requirement (for older people) of 0.91 protein/kg per day was calculated after reassessing data from three retrospective N-balance studies of older subjects and new data from Campbell et al. (*43*). In another study, older women were shown to adapt to marginal protein intakes (0.45 g protein/kg per day) by moving towards N equilibrium after 9 weeks. However, during this period there was a decline in lean tissue, immune response and muscle function. In the same study, women in N balance consuming 0.92 g protein/kg per day showed improvements in immune response and muscle function (*44*).

A3.5.3 **Disordered eating**

Disordered eating differs from established eating problems. In older adults, there may be an inappropriate sense of a need for weight change. However, excess fat for older people, although contributing to certain health problems, may be of less concern than a loss of lean mass. Factors contributing to disordered eating behaviour include prolongation of a minor eating disorder from earlier in life, preoccupation with the major morbidities and mortalities associated with later life, social isolation, physical handicaps, emotional difficulties and impaired cognitive function (*45, 46*).

A3.5.4 **Immune dysfunction**

The decline observed in immune function with ageing may be prevented with nutrient intakes greater than those currently recommended for normal health (*37*). Nutrients which are especially important in immune function include protein (*44, 47*), zinc (*48*), vitamin C, vitamin B6 and tocopherols (*49*). Other food components not usually considered to be essential for health may become so with age. For example, glutamine, which is a non-essential amino acid stored primarily in skeletal muscle (*50*), is utilized by intestinal cells, lymphocytes and macrophages, and is required for DNA and RNA synthesis (*51*). The rate of glutamine formation and availability can be compromised in older persons as a consequence of the reduced contribution of skeletal muscle to whole-body protein metabolism, thereby adversely affecting immune function and resulting in a less favourable response to infection or trauma (*51*). Glutamine can be synthesized from glutamic acid found in wheat, soybeans, lean meat and eggs. Glutathione (*52*) and flavonoids (*53*) also appear to play a role in immune function. Meat is a good source of glutathione, and moderate amounts are also found in fruits and vegetables. Whey proteins, although low in glutathione, are capable of stimulating endogenous glutathione production (*54*).

A3.5.5 *Cognitive impairment*

Long-term moderate (i.e. subclinical) nutrient deficiencies appear to contribute to memory impairment and declining immunity in older adults. On the other hand, dementia may result in nutritional deficiencies. Rosenberg & Miller (*41*) point to the growing evidence supporting the view that good nutritional status is an important determinant of quality of life because of its effect on the nervous system. For example, a healthy nervous system will maintain physical mobility, cognitive, psychological and visual function. Vitamins B6, B12 and C, and folate, riboflavin, thiamine and iron are needed for physical mobility and cognitive function (*55*). In a 20-year follow-up study of a community of older residents, cognitive function (independent of age, illness, social class or other dietary variables) was poorest in those persons with the lowest vitamin C status, whether measured by dietary intake or plasma ascorbic acid concentration (*56*). Vitamin K may also protect against cognitive decline and Alzheimer dementia (*57*).

Using the Mini-Mental State Examination and Pfeiffer's Mental Status Questionnaire developed by Folstein et al. (*58*), the cognitive status of a group of older adults from Madrid was found to be better in those consuming a more satisfactory diet (*59*), i.e. greater total food intake, especially of fruits and vegetables. Prevention of cognitive loss or dementia poses a particular challenge in older people. Some deterioration can be attributed to atherosclerotic disease and thus interventions such as aspirin usage or particular dietary patterns that reduce cardiovascular risk may also help prevent dementia.

A3.5.6 *Mood disturbance and depression*

There is a growing body of evidence suggesting that ω-3 polyunsaturated fatty acids play an important role in the etiology of depression (*60, 61*). Two studies have shown a positive correlation between the ratio of arachidonic acid to eicosapentaenoic acid (in plasma and erythrocyte membrane phospholipids) and the severity of depression (*62, 63*). In another study, a significant negative correlation was found between dietary ω-3 intake and the severity of depression (*64*). Fish and leafy vegetables (especially wild leafy greens) are a good source of ω-3 polyunsaturated fatty acids. Caffeine ingested either as tea or coffee has been shown to improve mood and reduce anxiety (*65*).

A3.6 **Developing food-based dietary guidelines for older adults**
A3.6.1 *The value of traditional cuisine*
It is clear that people of all nations and food cultures can enjoy comparable life expectancy and morbidity rates (*10, 40, 65*). The challenge lies in identifying those common food factors and patterns that reduce morbidity and mortality, thereby enabling the development of culture-specific food-based dietary guidelines that promote healthier traditional foods and dishes. Some adverse characteristics of traditional diets may have developed due to a lack of refrigeration and other food-preservation methods, or because of the limited availability of certain foodstuffs.

In the 1960s Greeks, followed by the Japanese, had the longest life expectancy in the world. The traditional Greek diet was associated with very low rates of coronary heart disease and cancers of the colon and breast (*17*). The intake of fish, legumes, cereals and alcohol in both countries was probably protective against coronary heart disease, whereas a high intake of salty foods/dishes contributed to increased risk of stroke and stomach cancer in Japan. Today the Japanese have the world's longest life expectancy, which has been attributed in part to their increased intake of fruit and fat and reduced intake of salty traditional dishes.

Prospective cohort studies conducted among older people in rural Greece (*67*), and in urban Australia (Melbourne) (*68*) and Denmark (Roskilde) (*69*), found that adherence to the traditional Greek food pattern was associated with lower overall mortality and longer survival. With a final score ranging between 0–8, the traditional Greek food pattern was rated in terms of eight variables: high consumption of vegetables; high consumption of legumes; high consumption of fruits; high consumption of cereals; low consumption of dairy products; low consumption of meat and meat products; moderate ethanol consumption; and a high mono-unsaturated: saturated fat ratio. A high score for the Greek food pattern was significantly associated with a sharply reduced risk of death, by 17–23% per one-unit increase and by more than 50% per four-unit increase in the different cultural settings. Whether further mortality benefit would have been obtained in the non-Greek cohorts if foods had been prepared according to Greek cuisine standards requires further study. Nevertheless, these studies suggest that the traditional Greek food pattern is transplantable to other dietary cultures and may have a substantial beneficial impact on the general mortality of older people with westernized dietary habits (*70*).

Traditional cuisines are often endangered cuisines because they are regarded as too old fashioned or time-consuming to prepare. With the submergence of traditional cuisines by other, more dominant, contemporary cuisines, we are increasingly witnessing a kind of culinary imperialism. This dilution of culture is occurring all over the world, especially in low-income countries (*71*). The younger generation, especially in urban regions of low-income countries, appears to be rejecting traditional foods in favour of western high-fat convenience foods (*72*). Whether this trend is correlated with anecdotal evidence that cooking skills are being lost, or that there is no time to cook, requires further investigation.

Multicultural Australia is a melting pot of culinary influences without a distinct Australian cuisine identity. However, Mediterranean and Asian cuisines are very popular. For example, the average Australian consumes Italian pasta dishes, pizza, and Asian stir-fry and noodle dishes throughout the week. Innovative Australian chefs are creating new dishes by combining the two cuisines where East meets West. It is forecast that the Eurasian cuisine developing in Australia and on the west coast of Canada and the USA will profoundly influence twenty-first century global cuisine. This has important implications for food-based dietary guidelines since it provides an opportunity to develop a super diet that includes the healthiest traditional foods and dishes from Asia and the Mediterranean region, and novel Eurasian dishes. The hope is that this will translate into longer and healthier lives for greater numbers.

A3.6.2 *Food habits of older persons, today and in the future*

Contrary to the popular tea and toast myth, it appears that most older persons residing outside of institutions eat reasonably well (*9, 40, 66, 73*). Energy intakes fall with advancing age, but average protein intakes remain adequate. The dietary patterns of older adults have generally been found to be similar to, or even healthier than, those of the younger generation (Table 1 and Table 2). Compared with their younger counterparts, and after controlling for energy intake, Australians aged 60 years and over were found in 1993 to have (*74*):

- A higher dietary density of breakfast cereals, breads and crackers (women only), fruit and fruit juice, vegetables, chicken, fish and eggs.
- A lower dietary density of rice and pasta, take-away foods and soft drinks.
- A similar dietary density of cakes, biscuits, confectionery, dairy, ice cream, processed meats, red meat, organ meats, spreads and sauces.

In contrast, in the USA there appears to be a stronger preference for sweets, cakes, pies, and some vegetables and fruits among older adults than in younger age groups (*79*). The analysis reported by Popkin et al. (*80*) indicates that older Americans have made dietary changes during the last decade that parallel those made by the rest of the population, i.e. a decreased intake of meat, and an increased intake of low-fat milk, low calorie beverages and take-away foods.

Some subgroups within older populations (e.g. older men living alone, those

Table 1.[a] **Mean daily food intakes of older Australians, compared to their middle-aged counterparts, in 1995[1]**

	65 and over		25–44 years		Recommended intake (g/day)[2]
	M	**F**	**M**	**F**	
N	**3337**	**2926**	**4189**	**3321**	
Cereals (e.g. rice, cakes)	200	150	230	170	> 210 g
Fruit (not juice)	179	176	127	132	300 g
Vegetables (not juice)	282	244	275	220	300–375 g
Milk products	340	300	390	300	450 g
Meat/poultry	146	95	212	121	85 g[3]
Fish & seafood	26	20	28	20	40 g[4]
Legumes (+ tofu)	9	3.6	11	8.4	> 30 g[4]
Nuts/seeds (e.g. peanut butter)	3	2	7	4	> 10 g[4]
Egg products	14	10	16	12	30 g or 2–4 eggs/ week
Snack foods (e.g. crisps)	0.8	0.4	4	4.4	
Sugar products (jam, sherbet)	28	17	22	14	
Confectionery (e.g. chocolate)	4	4	11	10	
Fats/oils	17	12	14	9	1–2 table- spoons (~30g)
Soup	77	69	40	53	
Savoury sauces	25	20	37	27	
Non-alcoholic beverages (e.g. tea, juice, water)	1644	1714	2162	2004	
Alcohol (pure)	15	5	20	8	men 20 g; women 10 g

[a] *Reproduced from reference 110 with the permission of the publisher.*

---

[1] Australian Bureau of Statistics (77).

[2] Cashel & Jefferson (75); Wahlqvist & Kouris-Blazos (76). Foods were converted to equivalents in core food groups as follows: 30 g bread is equivalent to 90 g cooked rice/ pasta or 20 g breakfast cereal; 150 g fruit is equivalent to one medium fruit (apple, orange, banana, 2 apricots, 1 cup diced pieces, edible portion); 75 g cooked vegetables is equivalent to 1/2 cup or 1 cup salad vegetables; 250 ml milk is equivalent to 1/2 cup evaporated milk or 40 g cheese or small tub (200 g) of yoghurt.

[3] In core food groups, 85 g/day of meat and meat equivalents are recommended. This includes red and white meat, eggs and legumes, e.g. 35 g cooked meat is equivalent to 40 g cooked fish fillet or 1/4 cup cooked beans or 1/3 cup nuts.

[4] Based on epidemiological studies of long-lived populations e.g. Greeks in Greece (Crete) in the 1960s, Greek-Australians, Japanese and vegetarians.

Table 2.[a] **Mean daily nutrient intakes of older Australians, compared to their middle-aged counterparts, in 1995[1]**

	65 and over		25–44 years		Recommended Intake[2]	
	M	**F**	**M**	**F**	**65+**	**19–64 years**
N	**3337**	**2926**	**4189**	**3321**		
Nutrients						
Energy kJ	8510	6370	11725	7875		
Protein % E	17	17.6	17	17	10–15	10–15
Total Fat % E	32	32	33	33	< 30	< 30
Saturated % E	2	12	13	13	< 10	< 10
Monounsaturated % E	11	11	12	12	10–15	10–15
Polyunsaturated % E	5	5	5	5	6–10	6–10
Carbohydrate % E	46	47	45	47	50–60	50–60
Total sugars % E	21	22	19	20	< 15	< 15
Total starch % E	25	26	26	26	40–50	40–50
Dietary fibre g	24	20	26	20	> 30	> 30
Alcohol % E	5	2	3	4	< 3	< 3
Vitamin A RE (µg)	1310	1064	1334	1038	750	750
Thiamin (mg)	1.6	1.2	2.1	1.4	0.9,0.7	1.1,0.8
Riboflavin (mg)	2.0	1.6	2.5	1.8	1.3,1.0	1.7,1.2
Niacin equivalent	39	39	54	35	16,11	19,13
Folate (mg)	280	225	311	227	200	200
Vitamin C (mg)	127	111	133	108	40,30	40,30
Calcium (mg)	796	686	990	762	800,1000	800
Phosphorus (mg)	1420	1132	1867	1300	1000	1000
Magnesium (mg)	334	268	392	284	320	320
Iron (mg)	14	11	17	12	7, 5–7	7, 12–6
Zinc	11	9	15	10	12	12
Potassium (mg)	3232	2626	3818	2816	1950–5460	1950–5460

[a] *Reproduced from reference 111 with the permission of the publisher.*

[1] Australian Bureau of Statistics (77).
[2] National Health & Medical Research Council (78); Wahlqvist & Kouris-Blazos (76).

with low socioeconomic status, the socially isolated, the institutionalized, the recently bereaved, the physically and socially inactive and the lonely) appear more likely to have inadequate diets (*9, 81–83*). Participation in fewer activities outside the home has also been linked to higher mortality in old age (*84*). In these subgroups there is greater risk of inadequate intakes of calcium, zinc, magnesium, vitamin B6 and folate (*9, 40, 74, 85*). Low intakes of these nutrients have important implications for bone health (calcium), wound healing (zinc), impaired immune response (zinc, vitamin B6) and vascular disease due to elevated homocysteine levels (folate). Other negative influences on dietary intake include physical disability, problems with chewing (loss of teeth and poorly fitting dentures), shopping difficulties and depression (*81*). Food-based dietary guidelines need to take account of the potential nutritional deficiencies that may occur in these subgroups.

Longitudinal changes (1988–1993) in the vitamin and mineral intakes of 2458 older Europeans born between 1913 and 1918 living in 18 towns in 12 countries (including the USA) were recently reported (*86*). In all towns, an increasing percentage of older adults did not meet the recommended nutrient densities and intakes for most nutrients (especially B vitamins, iron and calcium). This was accompanied by a reduced energy intake with 10% of the men and 30% of the women having energy intakes below 1500 kcal$_{th}$ (6.3MJ/day). The investigators concluded that older Europeans were at risk of malnutrition. In contrast, intakes of older Americans from the 1987–1988 National Food Consumption Survey were found to be adequate for most key nutrients. However, more detailed analyses are required to identify problem nutrients and the extent of deficient intakes in specific population subgroups (*79*). In particular the risks to the nutritional status of older persons in low-income and transitional countries need to be taken into consideration (*72, 85, 87*).

A3.6.3 *The demand for healthier fast foods*

Over the last decade, there has been a significant decline in the proportion of raw food grocery purchases in Australia. Simultaneously, the proportion of grocery expenditure on semi-prepared and high-convenience foods has increased considerably. In contrast to many low-income countries, a recent market survey of 1500 Australians aged 15 years and over found that the intake of high-fat western-style fast foods is on the decline. Australians are eating fewer hamburgers and less fried chicken and fried fish, and more fruit, vegetables and dairy products. Almost all consumers reported that fast food is fattening, suggesting changing preferences and an increasing demand for healthier fast foods.

High-fat fast foods have been replaced with healthier pre-packaged meals/ snacks—known as Meal Solutions or Home Meal Replacement—now available in supermarkets, and their heavy promotion is expected to have an impact on independent fast-food outlets. Changes in meal preparation from do it yourself to do it for me, where people are neglecting food preparation as part of daily life, have been attributed to time famine. As a result, new apartments are now being built in Australia and the USA without kitchens (*71, 88*). This trend, if confirmed, is likely to alter what people eat and thus have an impact on their health.

In contrast to younger adults, older persons are more likely to hold fast to traditional cuisines, including retention of cooking skills and a preference for home-cooked meals over take-away food (*72, 73, 89*). Studies in Japan indicate that older adults have a strong preference for low-fat traditional dishes containing fish and vegetables, and for traditional entrees as opposed to fast food, which tends to be higher in fat. However, preferences in Japan are expected to change since tomorrow's older person will have had greater exposure to higher-fat, non-traditional foods compared to today's (*89*). Food labels are diversifying rapidly and the market-place is replete with new products and the information that goes with them (*2*). Staying within one's traditional food culture may help to simplify nutritional decisions.

A recent market survey in Australia found that 34% of 1500 respondents reported buying freshly prepared take-away food from supermarkets during the previous 12 months, with younger people more likely to be purchasers of these foods. Market surveys are being conducted in Australia to determine to what extent older adults rely on pre-packaged meals from supermarkets and if there will be an increasing demand for them as the population ages. Ready-made meals for re-heating are reportedly widely used by older Europeans, while at the same time two-thirds of subjects consumed home-produced foods (*90*). This is an important signal for the processed-food industry that implies a multifaceted approach to nutrition in older adults. The use of convenience foods also confirms an earlier observation—that older adults introduce novel foods in their diet as often as younger adults do (*91*).

Should we be alarmed over the death of the family kitchen and loss of traditional cooking skills and recipes? Is it more rational to let the market supply many of these goods and services, especially for subgroups either who do not know how to cook or who cannot cook because of physical disabilities or lack of motivation, e.g. because they are living alone (*90*)? Time will tell. What is clear, however, is that if these trend forecasts are accurate they have important implications both for the development of food-based dietary guidelines and the role nutritionists and governments play in ensuring that consumers of all ages can make healthy choices when selecting pre-prepared foods (*79, 89*).

A3.6.4 *Nutrient needs*
Since older adults have reduced energy needs, they presumably receive lower amounts of the vitamins involved in energy metabolism. Lower energy needs are the result of a decline in metabolic rate (secondary to reduced lean muscle mass) and activity levels. Morbidity and mortality can be reduced in old age if lean body mass and physical activity are maintained at more youthful levels. The increased

food intake needed to balance a higher energy expenditure will help to ensure adequate intakes of essential nutrients. It is important that older adults with low-energy intakes consume nutrient-dense foods in preference to those with low nutrient density contributed by refined sugars, fats and alcohol.

Post-menopausal women have lower iron needs due to cessation of menstrual blood losses. However, chronic blood loss from gastrointestinal ulcers or other diseases, poor iron absorption or use of medications such as aspirin, which can cause blood loss, increase their risk of iron deficiency. Higher calcium requirements in estrogen-deprived post-menopausal women are reflected in recommendations for increased calcium intakes for this group.

There is also evidence that older persons have an increased need for vitamins B6, B12 and D, and a decreased need for vitamin A, than younger adults. In old age, the skin has a reduced capacity to synthesize previtamin D3, the kidneys experience impaired vitamin D3 hydroxylation and sun exposure tends to be reduced. Low serum vitamin A levels appear to be rare among older adults despite a high prevalence of dietary intakes below recommended levels (*9, 35, 92*). Trials of antioxidant vitamin supplementation (e.g. β-carotene, vitamin E) have shown no effect, or no adverse effect, in terms of cardiovascular disease, cancer or total mortality (*35*) that would justify increased intakes of these vitamins by older adults. Food-based dietary guidelines need to cover specifically ω-3 fats (α-linoleic acid, DHA and EPA) because of the role they are believed to play in:

- blood lipids (reduced triglycerides),
- blood clotting (reduced platelet aggregation),
- arthritis (reduced inflammation (*93, 94*)),
- depression (*61*), and
- abdominal obesity (*95*).

In summary, most older adults require the same intakes for most nutrients as younger adults, although this usually needs to be done through substantially lower overall food intakes. A nutrient-dense diet for older persons should thus be given high priority in any food-based dietary guidelines.

A3.6.5 *Process and implementation*
Designating a working group
An interdisciplinary, intersectoral working group or technical committee should undertake the development and implementation of food-based dietary guidelines. The expert advice of nutritionists and social scientists familiar with local culture and conditions is invaluable for identifying appropriate foods to promote and problems to avoid. Expertise beyond nutrition and public health should also be included, e.g. food science and technology, and the educational, behavioural, social, agricultural and environmental sciences (*96*).

Evaluating the major causes of morbidity and mortality and their dietary contributions within the older population

The process should begin with identifying relevant public health problems for older persons and determining the dietary and non-dietary factors that influence their incidence. More than simply identifying gaps between actual and recommended nutrient intakes, focusing on relevant public health problems requires an evaluation of the major causes of morbidity and mortality among older persons. As urban settings evolve, food-health relationships can be expected to vary as well, thereby requiring progressive reformulation of food-based dietary guidelines (*1*). Likely patterns of change include (*97*):

- increased rates of diabetes and ischaemic heart disease as modernization proceeds,
- a higher prevalence of obesity,
- the spread of fast-food outlets and an increase in food eaten outside the home, and
- increased fat consumption from foods eaten away from home.

Identifying foods, nutrients and phytochemicals associated with reduced morbidity and mortality in older adult

Once target nutrients and phytochemicals have been identified, a process should be implemented to identify appropriate foods for inclusion in food-based dietary guidelines. Information necessary for this analysis includes food choices permitting both high and low consumption of nutrients and phytochemicals, foods that are high in the selected nutrient or phytochemical, and the main dietary sources of these foods. The last group is not necessarily made up of foods with the highest nutrient concentrations, rather those that are most frequently consumed. The impact of these modifications on total nutrient and phytochemical profiles should also be considered.

Promoting healthy culture-specific traditional dishes and modern foods

Dietary advice that undermines trust in local cuisine, especially among people who have little manoeuvrability in terms of changing their practices, will be rejected or, worse still, diminish confidence in food selection and preparation (*98*). This impact can be of particular importance where food choices are changing under pressure of delocalization and globalization of the food supply (*99, 100*). Promoting traditional food choices and patterns is usually more effective than asking people to change their dietary habits. Assessing dietary intake, local cuisine, and food beliefs and practices to identify health-sustaining traditions is a good place to start promoting messages based on food-based dietary guidelines. Distinguishing traditional and modern foods/dishes as healthy or unhealthy can assist those responsible for developing food-based dietary guidelines at a time when dietary patterns are undergoing rapid change. Strategies to support retention of healthy traditions while encouraging healthy changes can be developed in this context.

Making sure that recommended foods/dishes are sustainable and do not harm the environment

Food-based dietary guidelines should accurately reflect a region's agricultural policies. Foods that are recommended in food-based dietary guidelines should be readily produced or obtained in the region without negative consequences for the environment or international trade.

Getting the message across to the target group

Food-based dietary guidelines should be developed in each country, and different sets may be required for specific geographic regions or socioeconomic groups within the same country. Food-based dietary guidelines should be seen within the broader community context. By combining information from different sources people may come up with quite a different message from the one health workers seek to promote. Thus, culturally appropriate models for presenting main messages should be sought, pre-tested, evaluated and revised before being disseminated widely.

A3.7 Principles governing food-based dietary guidelines for older adults

Probably the single most important health message for older persons is to achieve or maintain moderate levels of physical activity. There are similarities between the deterioration that occurs with ageing and that accompanying physical inactivity. Preventive measures to reduce diet-related disease should begin early in life, but it is never too late to start, even in old age. Given the behavioural risk factors (e.g. not eating breakfast, lack of regular physical activity, overweight and smoking) that have been shown to be predictors of 17-year mortality in individuals aged 70 and over, positive changes in lifestyle are worthwhile at every age.

Because older persons are more heterogeneous than any other age cohort, the individual's judgement plays a crucial role where acceptance of dietary and lifestyle changes is concerned. Physiological, psychological and sociological differences should thus be carefully considered. At one end of the spectrum are independent, vigorous and healthy people in their 70s, 80s and 90s. At the other are frail and dependent older persons with multiple diseases. Advice for the second group should probably focus mainly on function and quality of life rather than on diet or lifestyle.

There are five main ways to compress morbidity as near as possible to the end of life, and food-based dietary guidelines for older persons can help to promote all of them:

- Maintain social networks and social activity levels.
- Encourage physical activity throughout life.
- Discourage substance abuse.
- Encourage consumption of nutrient- and phytochemical-dense foods.
- Provide relevant, efficient and caring health services.

Each of these approaches requires sensitivity in culturally pluralistic societies and regions, as in the case of Australia and the Asia-Pacific Region generally.

The main nutritional factors to be considered in formulating food-based dietary guidelines for healthy ageing include:

- Food variety (*18, 20*) (Table 3).
- Nutrient density (*101*) (Table 4). Include culture-specific foods/dishes that are important sources of calcium, zinc, magnesium, vitamin B6, folate, vitamin D.
- Phytochemical density (*102, 103*) (Tables 5 and 6).

Fruits and vegetables can have special value for compressing morbidity (*104, 105*). High fruit and vegetable intakes have been most consistently associated with protection against macular degeneration, visual loss, cataracts, respiratory disease, and breast, stomach and colorectal cancer (*35*).

The minor components of cuisines, e.g. herbs and spices, may favourably influence health. For example, in older Greeks, a higher well-being and general health score and lower triglyceride concentrations were associated with a greater use of parsley, oregano and mint. Herbal tea (camomile, sage) was inversely related to abdominal fatness. Higher intakes of oregano and olive oil were associated with lower fasting blood glucose in subjects without diabetes (Kouris-Blazos et al., unpublished data).

Consumption of specific foods may also have a beneficial effect on health, e.g. fish (*14, 106*), lean meat (*76*), low-fat dairy products, tea (*107*), soy, legumes and nuts (*104, 108*), and unrefined fat from whole foods such as nuts, seeds and fatty fish. Where refined fats need to be used for cooking, it is preferable that they come from a variety of sources, including those that are high in ω-3 and ω-9 fats, i.e. canola, olives (preferably cold pressed or extra virgin) and soy bean. Fatty spreads should be avoided.

Food-based dietary guidelines may also need to consider the timing, frequency and size of meals for older adults. For example, in older Greeks, body fat mass has been negatively associated with greater meal/snack frequency, the consumption of two cooked meals daily, or when the main meal was taken at lunchtime and breakfast was eaten earlier rather than later in the morning.

Later dinner times were positively correlated with higher fasting blood glucose levels in people without diabetes. A more varied diet was positively associated

Table 3. **Weekly food variety score (1–57)**

Biologically distinct food groups	Score
1. Eggs (all varieties)	
DAIRY	//////
2. Milk, ice-cream, cheese	
LIVE CULTURES	//////
3. Yoghurt (e.g. acidophilus, bifidobacteria)	
YEAST	//////
4. Yeast extract	
FISH (+ canned)	//////
5. Fatty fish (tuna, anchovies, salmon, sardines, herring, mackerel, kipper)	
6. Saltwater fish	
7. Fresh-water fish	
8. Fish Roe (caviar salad)	
9. Shellfish (mussels, oysters, squid)	
10. Crustaceans (prawns, lobster)	
MEAT	//////
11. Ruminants (lamb, beef, veal)	
12. Monogastric (pork, ham, bacon)	
13. Poultry (chicken, duck, turkey)	
14. Game (quail, wild duck, pigeon)	
15. Game (kangaroo, rabbit)	
16. Liver	
17. Brain	
18. All other organ meats	
LEGUMES (+ canned)	//////
19. Peas (fresh, dried, split peas)	
Chickpeas (dried, roasted)	
Beans (haricot, kidney, lima, broad)	
Lentils (red, brown, green)	
Soy products (tofu, milk)	
CEREALS	//////
20. Wheat (bread, pasta, ready-to-eat)	
21. Corn (corn flakes, polenta)	
22. Barley (bread, barley cereal)	
23. Oats (porridge, cereal, bread)	
24. Rye (bread; ready-to-eat)	
25. Rice (grain, ready-to-eat)	
26. Other grains (millet, linseed)	
FATS & OILS	//////
27. Oils	
28. Hard/soft spreads	
BEVERAGES	//////
29. Tea, coffee, herbal teas	
30. Wine, beer, spirits	

Table 3. ***Weekly food variety score (1–57) (continued)***

Biologically distinct food groups	Score
FERMENTED FOODS	//////
31. Miso, tempeh, soy sauce	
32. Sauerkraut	
33. All other variety	
SUGAR/CONFECTIONERY	//////
34. All variety (+ soft drinks)	
VEGETABLES (+ canned, frozen)	//////
35. Root (potato, carrot, sweet potato, beetroot, parsnip, bamboo shoot, ginger, radish, water chestnut)	
36. Flowers (broccoli, cauliflower)	
37. Stalks (celery, asparagus)	
38. Onion (spring, garlic, leeks)	
39. Tomatoes, okra	
40. Beans (green, snow peas)	
41. Leafy greens (spinach, silverbeet, endive, kale, chicory, parsley, lettuce)	
42. Peppers (capsicum, chillies)	
43. Marrow (zucchini, squash, cucumber, turnip, eggplant, swede, pumpkin)	
44. Fungi (e.g. mushrooms)	
45. Herbs/spices	
NUTS & SEEDS	//////
46. Almond, cashew, chestnut, coconut, hazelnut, peanuts, peanut butter, pine nut, pistachio, pumpkin seed, sesame seed, tahini, walnut	
FRUIT	//////
47. Stone (peach, cherry, plums, apricot, avocado, olive, prune)	
48. Apples	
49. Pears, nashi	
50. Berries (strawberries)	
51. Grapes (and raisins, sultana)	
52. Bananas	
53. Citrus (orange, lemon)	
54. Melon (honeydew, watermelon)	
55. Kiwi, date, passion fruit	
56. Tropical (mango, pineapple)	
WATER	//////
57. Water (and mineral water)	
TOTAL WEEKLY VARIETY SCORE	

Instructions: A score of ONE is given to each food only ONCE if consumed (> 2 tablespoons) over a 7-day period. Score of biologically different foods consumed in a week: < 20 marginal; 20–24 fair; 25–29 good; > 30 very good.

[a] *Reproduced from reference 20 with the permission of the publisher.*

Table 4. **Nutrients, and good food sources for them, for which older persons are at risk of a deficiency**

Calcium	Milk and milk products, calcium-enriched soy products, salmon with bones, almonds, pulses, broccoli, tahini
Zinc	Lean red meat, liver, eggs, seafood, pork, nuts (e.g. cashews), pulses, whole grains, wheat germ, brewers yeast
Magnesium	Whole grains, seafood, soybeans, nuts, banana, avocado, pulses, salmon/tuna, meat, yoghurt, seeds
Vitamin B6	Common in foods, e.g. meats, liver, egg yolk, whole-grain cereals, pulses, yeast
Folate	Fresh leafy green vegetables, broccoli, oranges, avocado, yeast, liver, pulses, whole grain cereals, nuts
Vitamin D	Sardines, herring, salmon, cod-liver oil, egg yolks, butter, cheese

Adapted from: C.C. Horwath (81).

with alcohol consumption with dinner, and with a greater number of daily meals/snacks (3). Schlettwein-Gsell (109), who, using cross-sectional data, showed that older subjects most frequently ate regular meals, has hypothesized that this practice promotes a higher survival rate.

Many food components, once eaten, have detectable clinical effects. Although it may not always be known precisely which food components are responsible for which effects, there is good evidence that foods themselves, rather than isolated food components, are associated with good health. Thus, for example, a high intake of vegetables reduces the risk of many forms of cancer whereas isolating nutrients and taking them as a supplement does not appear to be protective. Moreover, certain food habits are associated with longevity e.g. those of Crete and Japan. This suggests that when it comes to health and longevity, the sum of the diet is greater than its individual parts; incorporating culture-specific cuisines into food-based dietary guidelines is therefore likely to result in a more favourable outcome than the incorporation of foods alone.

A3.8 **Summary and conclusion**

The main principles governing food-based dietary guidelines for older persons can be summarized as follows.

- Emphasize healthy traditional vegetable- and legume-based dishes where meat and nuts are used as condiments.
- Limit consumption of traditional dishes/foods that are heavily preserved/pickled in salt and encourage use of herbs and spices.

Table 5. **Food sources of phytochemicals and their possible roles in health**[a]

Phytochemicals	Some important food sources	Possible roles in health
Carotenoids	Orange pigmented, and green leafy vegetables, carrots, tomatoes, spinach	Antioxidant Antimutagen Anticarcinogen Immuno-enhancing
Flavonoids, isoflavonoids and saponins	Green and yellow leafy vegetables, parsley, celery, soybean and soy products	Antioxidant Anticarcinogen Estrogen Immuno-modulating
Polyphenolics	Cranberry, raspberries, blackberries, rosemary, oregano, thyme	Antioxidant Antibacterial Reduce urinary tract infection
Catechins	Green tea	Antimutagen Anticarcinogen Anticariogen
Isothiocyanates and indoles	Cruciferous vegetables, broccoli, cabbage	Antimutagen
Allyl sulphides	Garlic, onions, leeks	Anticarcinogen Antibacterial Cholesterol-lowering
Terpenoids including limonene	Citrus, caraway seeds	Anticarcinogenic against mammary tumours
Phytosterols	Pumpkin seeds	Reduce symptoms of prostate enlargement
Curcumin	Tumeric	Anti-inflammatory
Salicylates	Grapes, dates, cherries, pineapple, oranges, apricots, gherkins, mushrooms, capsicums, zucchini	Protective against macrovascular disease Modulation of gene expression
L-dopa	Broad bean	Treatment of Parkinson disease
Non-digestible carbohydrates	Artichoke, chicory root, murrnong, maize, garlic, oats, fruit, and vegetables	Stimulate growth of microbial flora Cholesterol-lowering

[a] *Reproduced from reference 3 with the permission of the publisher.*

Table 6. **Phytochemical-dense food checklist**[a]

This is not an exhaustive list of phytochemicals. Score 1 point for each food if eaten at least once a week, irrespective of serving size. If food is consumed more often, it still scores only one point.

Whole grains (unrefined) and cereals
- Barley
- Millet
- Rice
- Sorghum
- Maize/corn
- Oats
- Rye
- Wheat

Fruit
- Apples
- Apricots
- Other stone fruit, e.g. nectarines, peaches
- Berries, e.g. strawberries
- Citrus, e.g. orange, lemon, grapefruit
- Figs
- Currants and grapes, e.g. raisin, sultana
- Kiwi
- Melons
- Pears
- Paw-paw
- Other tropical fruit, e.g. mango, pineapple

Vegetables
- Artichoke
- Avocado
- Broccoli/cabbage/Brussels sprouts
- Sprouts/cauliflower
- Capsicum, red/green
- Carrots
- Cucumber
- Chili
- Fresh garlic
- Onions/leeks
- Potatoes
- Pumpkin
- Radish
- Rhubarb
- Swede

Vegetables (continued)
- Sweet potatoes
- Tomatoes
- Yams
- Dark-green leafy vegetables, e.g. spinach, endive, amaranth, silverbeet

Legumes/pulses
- Soy beans/soy products (tofu, soy milk)
- Chickpeas
- Lentils
- Peas
- Beans, e.g. kidney, halicot

Nuts and seeds
- Linseed
- Sesame seed
- Pumpkin seed
- Nuts
- Other nuts, e.g. peanuts, hazelnuts

Herbs and spices
- Basil
- Oregano
- Mint
- Dill/fennel
- Parsley
- Pepper
- Ginger
- Cumin
- Tumeric
- Coriander
- Rosemary/thyme

Beverages
- Fresh fruit juice
- Red wine
- Tea (green/black)

Oils
- Olive (unrefined)

[a] Reproduced from reference 20 with the permission of the publisher.

- Introduce healthy traditional foods or dishes from other cuisines (e.g. tofu into Mediterranean cuisines and the tomato into Asian cuisines) to increase the variety of foods consumed.

- Select nutrient-dense foods such as fish, lean meat, liver, eggs, soy products (e.g. tofu and tempeh) and low-fat dairy products, yeast or yeast-based products (e.g. spreads), fruits and vegetables, herbs and spices, whole-grain cereals, nuts and seeds.

- Consume fat from whole foods such as nuts, seeds, beans, olives and fatty fish. Where refined fats are used for cooking, select from a variety of liquid oils, including those that are high in ω-3 and ω-9 fats; avoid fatty spreads.

- Enjoy food and eating in the company of others, but avoid the regular use of celebratory foods (e.g. ice-cream, cakes and pastries in western food culture, confectioneries and candies in Malay food cultures and pork crackling in Chinese food culture).

- Encourage the processed-food industry and fast-food chains to make available—as alternatives to high-fat convenience foods—ready-made meals that are low in animal fats and high in nutrients and phytochemicals. The food industry can target older persons by developing a specific line of home-meal replacements fortified with the nutrients for which they are at greatest risk of deficiency. Food-based dietary guidelines can also include functional foods (e.g. bread based on whole grains and seeds such as soy and linseed).

- Several small non-fatty meals daily (5–6 eating episodes) appear to be associated with greater food variety and lower body fat, blood glucose and blood lipids, especially if food intake is curtailed in the evening hours. It is preferable to have the main meal at lunch and a light snack for dinner (3).

- As much as possible of one's food culture and health knowledge and related skills (e.g. regarding food production, choice, preparation and storage) should be transmitted both to one's children and grandchildren and to the broader community. Primary and secondary schools should be encouraged to teach all children about cooking as part of their practical survival skills.

- Older persons should be physically active on a regular basis and engage in exercises that strengthen muscles and improve balance. This will promote better energy (calorie) balance with weight maintenance, and more favourable body composition. It will also help to achieve adequate intake of nutrients and other food components since greater food intake is possible, without excessive energy intake, than would otherwise be possible with inactivity.

- To avoid dehydration, especially in warm climates, fluids should be drunk regularly and foods with a high water content eaten often.

Since these principles are to a degree technical in nature or have logistic implications, their application requires that local experts work with community elders in their implementation. As part of the new public health nutrition (*1*), whatever food-based dietary guidelines are developed should be subject to critical appraisal, monitoring and review, especially as regards their unintended consequences and ecological considerations.

The development of culturally sensitive food-based dietary guidelines, taking into account the best available scientific evidence, is preferable to advocating changes in food consumption patterns on the basis of studies of single food components and single disease outcomes.

Moreover, this approach is likely to result in fewer risks and greater benefits since many cultural food patterns have stood the test of time; in other words, they have been successfully established over many generations. There is still much to be distilled and learned from pooling the world's rich food-culture traditions and cuisines.

References

1. Wahlqvist ML et al. *Food-based dietary guidelines for the Western Pacific: the shift from nutrients and food groups to food availability, traditional cuisines and modern foods in relation to emergency chronic non-communicable diseases.* Manila, World Health Organization, Regional Office for the Western Pacific, 1999.

2. Wahlqvist ML et al. Nutrition in the 21st century: updates and challenges. In: Merican Z, Quee Lan Y eds. *Food agenda 21st century.* Malaysian Institute of Food Technology, Malaysia 1995:97–108.

3. Wahlqvist ML et al. Phytochemical deficiency disorders: inadequate intake of protective foods. *Current Therapeutics*, 1998, **39**:53–60.

4. Wahlqvist ML, Kouris-Blazos A, Hsu-Hage BH-H. Aging, food, culture and health. *Southeast Asian Journal of Tropical Medicine and Public Health*, 1997, **28** (Supple. 2):100–112.

5. Heikkinen E, Waters WE, Brezinski ZJ, eds. *The elderly in eleven countries—a sociomedical survey.* Copenhagen, World Health Organization, Regional Office for Europe, 1083 (Public Health in Europe Series, No. 21).

6. Butler R. Quality of life; can it be an endpoint? How can it be measured? *American Journal of Clinical Nutrition*, 1992, **55**:1267S–1270S.

7. Schlettwein-Gsell D. Nutrition and the quality of life: a measure for the outcome of nutritional intervention. *American Journal of Clinical Nutrition*, 1992, **55**:1263S–1266S.

8. Saltman D, Webster IW, Thernin GA. Older persons' definitions of good health: implications for general practitioners. *Medical Journal of Australia*, 1989, **150**:426–427.

9. Horwath CC. Nutrition and ageing. In: Mann JM, Truswell ST, eds. *Essentials of human nutrition.* New York, Oxford University Press, 1998:499–511.

10. *Preparation and use of food-based dietary guidelines: report of a joint FAO/WHO consultation.* Geneva, World Health Organization, 1998 (WHO Technical Report Series, No. 880).

11. Cassidy CM. Walk a mile in my shoes: culturally sensitive food-habit research. *American Journal of Clinical Nutrition*, 1994, **59** (Suppl.): 190S–197S.

12. McCully KS. Homocysteine and vascular disease. *Nature Medicine*, 1996, **2**:886–389.

13. Glueck CJ et al. Evidence that homocysteine is an independent risk factor for atherosclerosis in hyperlipidaemic patients. *American Journal of Cardiology*, 1995, **75**:132–136.

14. Kroumhout D, Bosschieter EBN, de Lesenne Coulander C. The inverse relation between fish consumption and 20-year mortality from coronary heart disease. *New England Journal of Medicine*, 1985, **312**:1205–1209.

15. Kroumhout D, Fedkens EJM, Bowles CH. The protective effect of a small amount of fish on coronary heart disease mortality in an elderly population. *International Journal of Epidemiology*, 1995, **24**:340–345.

16. Hertog MG et al. Dietary antioxidant flavonoids and risk of coronary heart disease: the Zutphen elderly study. *Lancet*, 1993, **342**:340–345.

17. Willet W. Diet and health: what should be eat? *Science*, 1994, **264**:532–537.

18. Hodgson JM, Hsu-Hage BH-H, Wahlqvist ML. Food variety as a quantitative descriptor of food intake. *Ecology of Food and Nutrition*, 1994, **32**:137–148.

19. Hsu-Hage BH-H, Wahlqvist ML. Food variety of adult Melbourne Chinese: a case study of a population in transition. *World Review of Nutrition and Dietetics*, 1996, **79**:53–69.

20. Savige GS, Hsu-Hage BH-H, Wahlqvist ML. Food variety as nutritional therapy. *Current Therapeutics*, **38**:57–67.

21. Tontisirin K, Kosulwat V. National dietary guidelines: current status and application in Asian countries. In: *Dietary guidelines in Asian countries: towards a food-based approach*. Florentino RF, ed. Washington, DC, International Life Sciences Institute, 1997:13–20.

22. Sakamoto M. Nutrient needs through the life cycle. In: *Dietary guidelines in Asian countries: towards a food-based approach*. Florentino RF, ed. Washington, DC, International Life Sciences Institute, 1997:43–49.

23. Darnton-Hill I, de Boer A, Nishida C. Overview of nutrition in the Western Pacific Region of the World Health Organization. *Australian Journal of Nutrition and Diet*, 1996, **53**: 171–174.

24. Murray CJL, Lopez AD. *Summary: the global burden of disease and injury*. Boston, MA, Harvard School of Public Health, 1996.

25. Khor GL. Nutrition and cardiovascular disease: an Asian-Pacific perspective. *Asia Pacific Journal of Clinical Nutrition*, 1997: **6**:122–142.

26. *Diet, nutrition and the prevention of chronic diseases*. Geneva, World Health Organization, 1990 (WHO Technical Report Series, No. 797).

27. Buskirk ER. Health maintenance and longevity: exercise. In: Finch CE & Schneider EL, eds. *The handbook of biology and ageing*. New York, Van Nostrand Reinhold, 1985:894–931.

28. Fries JF. Physical activity, the compression of morbidity, and the health of the elderly. *Journal of the Royal Society of Medicine*,1996, **89**:64–68.

29. Astrand PO. Physical activity and fitness. *American Journal of Clinical Nutrition*, 1992, **55**: 1231S–1236S.

30. Kushi L et al. Diet and 20-year mortality from coronary heart disease. The Ireland-Boston Diet Heart Study. *New England Journal of Medicine*, 1985, **312**:811–818.

31. Lapidus L, Bengtsson C. Socioeconomic factors and physical activity in relation to cardiovascular disease and health. A 12 year follow-up of participants in a population study of women in Gothenburg, Sweden. *British Heart Journal*, 1986, **55**:295–301.

32. Morris JN, Marr JW, Clayton DG. Diet and heart: a postscript. *British Medical Journal*, 1977, **2**:1307–1314.

33. Kromhout D, Bosschieter EB, de Lezenne Coulander C. Dietary fibre and 10-year mortality for coronary heart disease, cancer and all causes. *Lancet*, 1984, **2**:518–521.

34. Paffenbarger RS et al. The association of changes in physical-activity level and other lifestyle characteristics with mortality among men. *New England Journal of Medicine*, 1993; **328**:538–545.

35. Khaw KT. Healthy ageing. *British Medical Journal*, 1997, **315**:1090–1096.

36. Fiatarone MA et al. Exercise training and nutritional supplementation for physical frailty in very elderly people. *New England Journal of Medicine*, 1995, **330**:1769–1775.

37. Chandra RK. Effect of vitamin and trace-element supplementation on immune responses and infection in elderly subject. *Lancet*, 1992, **340**:1124–1127.

38. Lukito W, Boyce NW, Chandra RK. Nutrition and Immunity. In: Wahlqvist ML, Vobecky JS, eds. *The Medical Practice of Preventive Medicine*. London, Smith-Gordon & Co Ltd., 1994:27–51.

39. Schroll M, Aylund K, Davidsen M. Predictors of five-year functional ability in a longitudinal survey of men and women aged 75 to 80. The 1914 population in Glostrup, Denmark. *Ageing* 1997; **9**:143–152.

40. Wahlqvist ML et al., eds. Food habits in later life: a cross-cultural study. Melbourne: *Asia Pacific Journal of Clinical Nutrition* & United Nations University Press, 1995 (CD-ROM).

41. Rosenberg IH, Miller J. Nutritional factors in physical and cognitive functions of elderly people. *American Journal of Clinical Nutrition*, 1992; **55**:1237S–1243S.

42. Chumlea WC et al. Techniques of assessing muscle mass and function (sarcopenia) for epidemiological studies of the elderly. *Journal of Gerontology*, 1995, 50A, Special No.: 45–51.

43. Campbell WW et al. Increased protein requirements in elderly people: new data and retrospective assessments. *American Journal of Clinical Nutrition*, 1994, **60**:501–509.

44. Castaneda C et al. Elderly women accommodate to a low-protein diet with losses of body cell mass, muscle function, and immune response. *American Journal of Clinical Nutrition*, 1995, **62**:30–39.

45. Wahlqvist ML, Russell J, Beumont P. Prevention of dieting disorders: screening and preventive intervention (the NHMRC initiative). *Asia Pacific Journal of Clinical Nutrition*, 1997; **6**:153–161.

46. Clarke DM et al. Psychological factors in nutritional disorders of the elderly: Part of the spectrum of eating disorders. *International Journal of Eating Disorders*, 1999, **25**:345–348.

47. Chandra RK et al. Nutrition and immunocompetence of the elderly: effects of short-term nutritional supplementation on cell-mediated immunity and lymphocyte subsets. *Nutrition Research*, 1982, **2**:223–232.

48. Chandra RK, McBean LD. Zinc and immunity. *Nutrition*, 1994, **1**:79–80.

49. Grimble RF. Effects of antioxidative vitamins on immune function with clinical applications. *International Journal of Vitamin and Mineral Research*, 1997, **67**:312–320.

50. Newsholme EA. The possible role of glutamine in some cells of the immune system and the possible consequence for the whole animal. *Experientia*, 1996; **52**:455–459.

51. Young VR. Amino acids and proteins in relation to the nutrition of elderly people. *Age and Ageing*. 1990; **19**:10S–24S.

52. Jones DP et al. Glutathione in foods listed in the National Cancer Institute's Health Habits and History Food Frequency Questionnaire. *Nutrition and Cancer*, 1992, **17**:57–75.

53. Middleton E Jr, Kandaswami C. Effects of flavonoids on immune and inflammatory cell functions. *Biochemical Pharmacology*, 1992, **43**:1167–1179.

54. Regester GO. *Whey protein based functional foods*. Proceedings of an International Workshop on functional foods—the present and the future. Canberra, National Food Authority, 5–6 Oct 1993.

55. Goodwin JS, Goodwin JM, Garry PJ. Association between nutritional status and cognitive functioning in a healthy elderly population. *Journal of the American Medical Association*, 1983, **249**:2917–2921.

56. Gale CR, Martyn CN, Cooper C. Cognitive impairment and mortality in a cohort of elderly people. *British Medical Journal*, 1996, **312**:608–611.

57. Kohlmeier M. Interaction of the apolipoprotein E4 allele and vitamin K status—A possible role in the development of cognitive decline and Alzheimer's dementia. In: Andrews GR et al, eds. *Ageing beyond 2000: One world one future*. Book of abstracts. Bedford Park, South Australia, World Congress of Gerontology, 1997:3.

58. Folstein MF, Folstein SE, McHugh PR."Mini-mental state". A practical method for grading the cognitive state of patients for the clinician. *Journal of Psychiatric Research*, 1975; **2**:189–198.

59. Ortega RM et al. Dietary intake and cognitive function in a group of elderly people. *American Journal of Clinical Nutrition*, 1997; **66**:803–809.

60. Hibbeln JR, Salem N. Dietary polyunsaturated fatty acids and depression: when cholesterol does not satisfy. *American Journal of Clinical Nutrition*, 1995, **62**:1–9.

61. Peet M, Edwards RW. Lipids, depression and physical disease. *Current Opinion in Psychiatry* 1997; **10**:477–480.

62. Maes M et al. Fatty acid composition in major depression: decreased omega 3 fractions in cholesteryl esters and increased C20: 4 omega 6/C20:5 omega 3 ratio in cholesteryl esters and phospholipids. *Journal of Affective Disorders*, 1996, **38**:35–46.

63. Adams PB et al. Arachidonic acid to eicosapentanoic acid ratio in blood correlates positively with clinical symptoms of depression. *Lipids*, 1996, **31**:157S–161S.

64. Edwards RH et al. Omega-3 polyunsaturated fatty acid levels in the diet and in red blood cell membranes of depressed patients. *Journal of Affective Disorders*, 1998, **48**:149–155.

65. Quinlan P, Lane J, Aspinall L. Effects of hot tea, coffee and water ingestion on physiological responses and mood—the role of caffeine, water and beverage type. *Psychopharmacology*, 1997; **134**:164–173.

66. Wahlqvist ML et al. Food habits in later life—an overview of key findings. *Asia Pacific Journal of Clinical Nutrition*, 1995; **4**:1–11.

67. Trichopoulou A et al. Diet and overall survival in elderly people. *British Medical Journal*, 1995; **311**:1457–1460.

68. Kouris-Blazos A et al. Are the advantages of the Mediterranean diet transferable to other populations? A cohort study in Melbourne, Australia. *British Journal of Nutrition*, 1999, **82**:57–61.

69. Osler M, Schroll M. Diet and mortality in a cohort of elderly people in a north European community. *International Journal of Epidemiology*, 1997; **26**:155–159.

70. Kouris-Blazos A, Wahlqvist ML. The traditional Greek food pattern and overall survival in elderly people. *Australian Journal Nutrition and Diet*, 1998, **55** (Suppl. 4):20–24.

71. Ripe C. *Goodbye culinary cringe*. Sydney, Allen & Unwin, 1993.

72. Wahlqvist ML, Lukito W, Hsu-Hage BH-H. Nutrition and Ageing in Development. In: Biswas MR, Gabr M, eds. *Nutrition in the 90s—policy issues*. Oxford, Oxford University Press, 1994:84–108.

73. Kouris-Blazos A et al. Health & Nutritional Status of elderly Greek migrants to Melbourne, Australia. *Age and Ageing*, 1996, **25**:177–189.

74. CSIRO. *Does five years make a difference? Results from Australian food and nutrition surveys 1998 and 1993*. Clayton South VIC 3169, Australia, Commonwealth Scientific & Industrial Research Organisation, Division of Human Nutrition, 1996.

75. Cashel K, Jefferson S. *The core food groups. The scientific basis for developing nutrition education tools*. National Health & Medical Research Council, Canberra, Australian Government Publishing Service, 1995.

76. Wahlqvist ML, Kouris-Blazos A. Dietary Advice and Food Guidance Systems. In: Wahlqvist ML, ed. *Food and nutrition: Australia, Asia and the Pacific.* Sydney, Allen & Unwin, 1997:508–522.

77. Australian Bureau of Statistics. *National Nutrition Survey Selected Highlights.* Melbourne, Australia, 1994. Canberra, Australian Government Publishing Service, 1997.

78. National Health & Medical Research Council. *Recommended dietary intakes for use in Canberra.* Canberra, Australian Government Publishing Service, 1991.

79. Dichter CR. Designing foods for the elderly: an American view. *Nutrition Reviews*, 1992, **50**:480–483.

80. Popkin BM, Haines PS, Patterson RE. Dietary changes in older Americans, 1977–1987. *American Journal of Clinical Nutrition* 1992; **55**:823–830.

81. Horwath CC. Dietary intake studies in elderly people. In: Bourne GH, ed. Impact of nutrition on health and disease. *World Review of Nutrition and Diet*, 1989, **59**:1–70.

82. Horwath CC. Socioeconomic and behavioural effects of the dietary habits of elderly people. *International Journal of Biosocial and Medical Research*, 1989, **11**:15–30.

83. SENECA Investigators. Dietary habits and attitudes. *European Journal of Clinical Nutrition* 1991; **45**:83–95.

84. Olsen RB et al. Social networks and longevity. A 14-year follow-up study among elderly in Denmark. *Social Science and Medicine*, 1991; **33**:1189–1195.

85. Wahlqvist ML et al. Water-soluble vitamin intakes in the elderly: cross-cultural findings in the IUNS study. In: *Nutritional assessment of elderly populations: measure and function.* Rosenberg IH, ed. New York, Raven Press, 1994:225–233.

86. SENECA Investigators. Longitudinal changes in the intake of vitamins and minerals of elderly Europeans. *European Journal of Clinical Nutrition* 1996; **50**:77–85.

87. Pongpaew P, Schelp FP. Elderly in a country going through epidemiological health transition—the example of Thailand. *Age & Nutrition* 1997; **8**:30–35.

88. Sidler H. Meal Solutions. *Nutrition News: National Heart Foundation.* Issue 25, 1998:6.

89. Fukuba H. Meeting the challenges of an ageing population: an overview. *Nutrition Reviews*, 1992, **50**:467–471.

90. Hautvast JGAJ et al. How food-related industries can respond to the nutritional needs of the elderly: a European view. *Nutrition Reviews*, 1992, **50**:484–487.

91. Davies L. *Three score years ..... and then? A study of the nutrition and well-being of elderly people at home.* London, Heinemann, 1981.

92. Russell RM. Micronutrient requirements of the elderly. *Nutrition Reviews* 1992; **50**:463–466.

93. Nettleton JA. *Omega-3 fatty acids in health.* New York, Chapman & Hall, 1995.

94. James M., Cleland LG. Dietary n-3 fatty acids and therapy for rheumatoid arthritis. *Seminars in Arthritis and Rheumatism*, 1997, **27**:85–89.

95. Couet C et al. Effect of dietary fish oil on body fat mass and basal fat oxidation in healthy adults. *International Journal of Obesity*, 1997, **21**:637–643.

96. Schneeman BO. Food Based Dietary Guidelines. In: *Dietary guidelines in Asian countries: Towards a food-based approach.* Florentino RF, ed. Washington, DC, International Life Sciences Institute, 1997:9–12.

97. Binns CW. Dietary guidelines for optimal health: A checklist and a few hints. In: Florentino RF ed. *Dietary guidelines in Asian countries: towards a food-based approach.* Washington, DC, International Life Sciences Institute, 1997:39–42.

98. Sellerberg M. In food we trust? Vitally necessary confidence—and untraditional ways of attaining it. In: Furst EL et al., eds. *Palatable worlds: Sociocultural food studies*. Oslo, Solum Forlag, 1991:193–202.

99. Pelto GH, Pelto PJ. Diet and Delocalisation: Dietary Changes since 1750. In: Rotberg R, Rabb T, eds. *Hunger and history: The impact of changing food production and consumption patterns on society*. Cambridge, Cambridge University Press, 1985:309–330.

100. Pelto PJ, Pelto GH. Studying knowledge, culture and behaviour in applied medical anthropology. *Medical Anthropology Quarterly*, 1997; **11**:147–163.

101. Wahlqvist ML, Flint DM. Nutrition requirements and recommended dietary intakes for the elderly—Vitamins. In: *Nutrition in the elderly*. Washington, DC, World Health Organization, Regional Office for the Americas, Oxford University Press, 1989:123–136.

102. Wahlqvist ML, Kouris-Blazos A, Watanapenpaiboon N. The significance of eating patterns: an elderly Greek case study. *Appetite*, 1998; **32**:1–10.

103. Wahlqvist ML, Dalais F. Phytoestrogens—the emerging multifaceted plant compounds. (Editorial) *Medical Journal of Australia*, 1997; **167**:119–120.

104. Kant AK et al. Dietary diversity and subsequent mortality in the First National Health and Nutrition Examination Survey Epidemiologic Follow-up Study. *American Journal of Clinical Nutrition*, 1993, **57**:434–440.

105. Wahlqvist ML. Nutritional factors in carcinogenesis. *Asia Pacific Journal of Clinical Nutrition*, 1993; **2**:141–148.

106. Wahlqvist ML. Fish and human health. Food and Nutrition Conference, Surabaya, Indonesia, 9–10 December 1996.

107. Yang CS. Tea and cancer (review). *Journal of the National Cancer Institute*, 1993; **85**:1038–1049.

108. Dreher ML, Maher CV, Kearney P. The traditional and emerging role of nuts in healthful diets. *Nutrition Reviews*, 1996; **54**:241–245.

109. Schlettwein-Gsell D. Zur Ernährungssituation der Betagten. [On the nutrition situation of the elderly]. In: Aebi H et al., eds. 2. *Schweizerische Ernahrungsbericht [Swiss Nutrition Review]*. Bern, Hans Huber, 1984:262–272.

110. Wahlqvist ML, Kouris-Blazos A. Requirements in maturity and ageing. In: Wahlqvist ML, ed. *Food and Nutrition: Australia and New Zealand*, 2nd ed. Sydney, Allen & Unwin, 2002:348.

111. Wahlqvist ML, Kouris-Blazos A. Requirements in maturity and ageing. In: Wahlqvist ML, ed. *Food and Nutrition: Australia and New Zealand*, 2nd ed. Sydney, Allen & Unwin, 2002:350.

The Heidelberg guidelines for promoting physical activity among older persons*

Target: older persons

Physically active lifestyles benefit individuals throughout the life span. These guidelines were however developed primarily for promoting physical activity in the latter half of the life course. Although much of their content equally applies to individuals in other age groups, the scientific committee in charge of developing these guidelines selected those aged 50 years and above as the most appropriate target.

Age 50 marks a point in middle age at which the benefits of regular physical activity can be most relevant in avoiding, minimizing, and/or reversing many of the physical, psychological, and social problems which often accompany advancing age. These beneficial effects apply to most individuals regardless of health status and/or disease state.

Within these guidelines, physical activity is operationally defined as all movements in everyday life, including work, activities of daily living, recreation, exercise, and sporting activities. The proposed guidelines recognize that the preventative and rehabilitative effects of regular physical activity are optimized when physical activity patterns are adapted early in life, rather than when initiated in old age.

The guidelines focus on the impact of regular physical activity for both sexes. However, due to historical differences in the prevalence of physically activity lifestyles between the sexes, as well as the greater proportion of women in the older adult population, the scientific committee is careful to emphasize that the guidelines are universal and apply equally to all. Similarly, it is also clear that the guidelines must be sufficiently flexible to be of meaning to a wide variety of social and cultural groups.

The aim is to provide guidelines for facilitating the development of strategies and policies in both population and community-based interventions aimed at maintaining and/or increasing the level of physical activity for all older adults.

---

* These Guidelines were prepared by a scientific committee, submitted to participants at the 4th International Congress on Physical Activity, Ageing and Sports (Heidelberg, Germany, August 1996) and finalized by the World Health Organization.

http://www.who.int/hpr/ageing/heidelberg_eng.pdf

Evidence

Appropriate physical activity can be fun and is good for you!

Most people who engage in recreational physical activity do so because it is fun and enjoyable. Furthermore, there is ample evidence to show that physical activity is associated with significant improvements in functional ability and health status and may frequently prevent certain diseases or diminish their severity. However, it is important to note that many of these benefits require regular and continuous participation and can be rapidly reversed by a return to inactivity.

Scientific evidence has shown that regular physical activity:

- Enhances general well-being
- Improves overall physical and psychological health
- Helps to preserve independent living
- Reduces the risk of developing certain noncommunicable diseases (e.g. CHD, hypertension, etc.)
- Helps in the control of specific conditions (e.g. stress and obesity) and diseases (e.g. diabetes and hypercholesterolaemia)
- Helps to minimize the consequences of certain disabilities and can help in the management of painful conditions
- May help change stereotypic perspectives of old age

Benefits of physical activity for the individual
Immediate physiological benefits

- *Glucose levels*: Physical activity helps regulate blood glucose levels.
- *Catecholamine activity*: Both adrenaline and noradrenaline levels are stimulated by physical activity.
- *Improved sleep*: Physical activity has been shown to enhance sleep quality and quantity in individuals of all ages.

Long-term physiological benefits

- *Aerobic/cardiovascular endurance*: Substantial improvements in almost all aspects of cardiovascular functioning have been observed following appropriate physical training.
- *Resistive training/muscle strengthening*: Individuals of all ages can benefit from muscle strengthening exercises. Resistance training can have a significant impact and the maintenance of independence in old age.
- *Flexibility*: Exercise, which stimulates movement throughout the range of motion, assists in the preservation and restoration of flexibility.

- *Balance/coordination*: Regular activity helps prevent and/or postpone the age-associated declines in balance and coordination that are a major risk factor for falls.

- *Velocity of movement*: Behavioural slowing is a characteristic of advancing age. Individuals who are regularly active can often postpone these age-related declines.

Immediate psychological benefits

- *Relaxation*: Appropriate physical activity enhances relaxation.

- *Reduces stress and anxiety*: There is evidence that regular physical activity can reduce stress and anxiety.

- *Enhanced mood state*: Numerous people report improvement in mood state following appropriate physical activity.

Long-term psychological effects

- *General well being*: Improvements in almost all aspects of psychological functioning have been observed following periods of extended physical activity.

- *Improved mental health*: Regular exercise can make an important contribution in the treatment of several mental illnesses, including depression and anxiety neurosis.

- *Cognitive improvements*: Regular physical activity may help postpone age related declines in Central Nervous System processing speed and improve reaction time.

- *Motor control and performance*: Regular activity helps prevent and/or postpone the age-associated declines in both fine and gross motor performance.

- *Skill acquisition*: New skills can be learned and existing skills refined by all individuals regardless of age.

Immediate social benefits

- *Empowering older individuals*: A large proportion of the older adult population gradually adopts a sedentary lifestyle, which eventually threatens to reduce independence and self-sufficiency. Participation in appropriate physical activity can help empower older individuals and assist them in playing a more active role in society.

- *Enhanced social integration*: Physical activity programmes, particularly when carried out in small groups and/or in social environments enhance social and intercultural interactions for many older adults.

Long-term social effects

- *Enhanced integration*: Regularly active individuals are less likely to withdraw from society and more likely to actively contribute to the social milieu.

- *Formation of new friendships*: Participation in physical activity, particularly in small groups and other social environments stimulates new friendships and acquaintances.

- *Widened social networks*: Physical activity frequently provides individuals with an opportunity to widen available social networks.

- *Role maintenance and new role acquisition*: A physically active lifestyle helps foster the stimulating environments necessary for maintaining an active role in society, as well as for acquiring positive new roles.

- *Enhanced intergenerational activity*: In many societies, physical activity is a shared activity, which provides opportunities for intergenerational contact thereby diminishing stereotypic perceptions about ageing and older persons.

Benefits for society

- *Reduced health and social care costs*: Physical inactivity and sedentary living contributes to a decrease in independence and the onset of many chronic diseases. Physically active lifestyles can help postpone the onset of physical frailty and disease thereby significantly reducing health and social care costs.

- *Enhancing the productivity of older adults*: Older individuals have much to contribute to society. Physically active lifestyles help older adults maintain functional independence and optimize the extent to which they are able to actively participate in society.

- *Promoting a positive and active image of older persons*: A society which promotes a physically active lifestyle for older adults is more likely to reap the benefits of the wealth of experience and wisdom possessed by the older individuals in the community.

Who should be physically active?

Regular physical activity has significant physical, psychological, social and cultural benefits for individuals of all ages, including those with specific limitations and disabilities.

There are individuals and groups with special needs who may have particular requirements which will have to be met in order to optimize the effectiveness of both acute and long term physical activity (e.g. need for special access, reduction of environmental obstacles, modified programmes and equipment). Implementation strategies, policies, and educational programmes must take into consideration the exceptional needs and requirements of these populations.

Figure 1. **Health–fitness gradient**

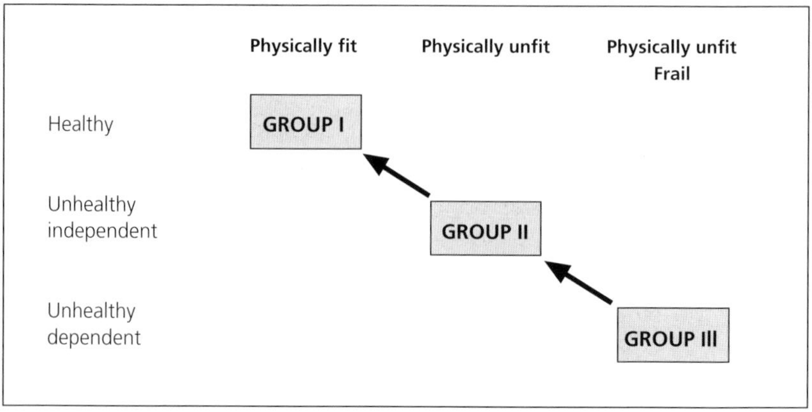

Specific physical activity needs will vary as a function of the individual's position along a Health–fitness gradient (Figure 1).

Group One: Physically fit—healthy:
These individuals regularly engage in appropriate physical activity, they can be described as physically fit and can participate in all activities of daily living.

Group Two: Physically unfit—unhealthy independent:
These individuals are not engaged in physical activity. While they are still living independently, they are beginning to develop multiple chronic medical conditions that threaten their independence. Regular physical activity can help improve functional capacity and prevent loss of independence.

Group Three: Physically unfit frail—unhealthy dependent:
These individuals are no longer able to function independently in society due to a variety of physical and/or-psychological reasons. Appropriate physical activity can significantly enhance the quality of life and restore independence in some areas of functioning.

Promoting and facilitating increased physical activity

There is a need to stimulate greater appreciation for the importance of regular physical activity among policy makers at all levels of administration:

- International
- National
- Regional
- Local

Educating, disseminating, and creating conductive environments

There is also a need to involve a wide variety of sectors in the dissemination of information on healthy ageing and in supporting favourable environments in the promotion of physical activity, such as:

- Family support
- Peer-support groups (e.g. national councils on ageing).
- Community and social service providers
- The media
- Nongovernmental organizations
- Self-help groups
- Health care providers
  — Primary care team
  — Hospital
  — Nursing home
  — Health insurers
- Universities
- Adult education institutions
- Rehabilitation and therapeutic centres
- Residential facilities
- Private and public sector organizations (e.g. workplace)
- Sporting and social clubs

Implementing physical activity
The setting: facilitating increased physical activity

There is a need to develop strategies that will lead to increased levels of physical activity throughout all segments of the population. Such a healthy public policy can only be achieved by influencing:

Health policy

- It is not necessary to have expensive facilities and equipment.
- Physical activity can be effective in environments with limited space and resources (e.g. home environments).
- The workplace can be an appropriate site for providing physical activity programmes.

Safety issues

- Medical advice may be desirable for some individuals before beginning an activity programme.

- Appropriately training at all levels (participants, trainers, programme planners and evacuators) is recommended.
- Safe environments are important (e.g. adequate lighting, ramps).
- It is important to reduce environmental obstacles.

Motivating factors
- Physical activity can be fun
- Companionship
- Enhanced control over one's own life
- Lifelong activity (sport biography)
- Improved health status and well-being

The barriers among primary caregivers and other health service providers in society
- Stereotypical images of ageing
- Low social support
- Inadequate environmental support for physical activity (e.g. transportation, access, urban planning)
- Life history/biographical aspects, including bad experiences with sports
- Negative attitudes towards sports and exercise
- Imbalance of expected effort and perceived gains
- Social obstacles towards a healthy lifestyle
- Inappropriate social and cultural settings

Certain medical conditions may require modified activity programmes.

Types of physical activity

Many individuals have a physically active lifestyle without necessarily participating in formal exercise programmes. Through usual activities of daily living, e.g. working, shopping, cooking and cleaning etc., one can maintain an adequate level of activity, even without a high degree of aerobic performance. The first message to be given to individuals as they age is that they should be active in their everyday life. However, in industrialized societies, lifestyles are often associated with a level of physical activity below adequate levels.

Structured activity programmes provide ways for individuals to promote a physically active lifestyle. The recommendations for these programmes include:

- Individual and/or group activity need not necessarily be performed in supervised settings.

- There are benefits associated with various types of physical activity including stretching, relaxation, callisthenics, aerobic exercise, and strength training among others.
- The focus should be on simple and moderate forms of physical activity (e.g. walking, dancing, stair climbing, swimming, cycling, chair exercises, etc.).
- Important components to consider in an exercise programme include aerobic exercise, muscular strength, flexibility, and balance.
- Exercise must meet individual and group needs and expectations.
- Exercise should be relaxing and enjoyable. Have fun!
- Exercise should be regular, if possible daily.

Research

Additional research for the promotion of physical activity in older persons is required. This implies appropriate levels of funding. Research of special interest includes outcome assessment and evaluation of interventions that reflect the different dimensions specific in these guidelines.

BOOK